Advanced Praise for
The Supercharged Method

"Starting from high school I feel like I've spent my entire life reading diet and health books. I didn't think anything could teach me or surprise me anymore—until now. I challenge you to open *The Supercharged Method* to any page and read it while you're standing there in the bookstore aisle. I bet you there's not a single page that won't tell you something you didn't know and find of value to both your body and mind. Doctor Francis has done a stellar job of synthesizing her years of study and research. Take advantage of her knowledge and practice."

—Andrew Lebby, PhD, Founding Partner,
The Performance Group, Washington, DC

"This book is for anyone who's confusion of how to start on a new path has led to inaction. It's written in a very easy to approach manner. Humor and simple steps make this a must have for anyone stuck in a rut, not knowing which direction to turn. Many lives will be changed with this book, it's time to make yours one of them."

—Dr. Jennifer Shell, Chiropractor, essential oil expert,
and author of *Food to the Rescue*

D1478199

"Encouraging self care is really the crux of this book. We must prioritize ourselves and our health, and in doing so we also become better support for others. Overall, I found *The Supercharged Method* to be straightforward, easy to understand, relatable, and able to meet people where they are at, without judgment. Dr. Francis covers so much in this book, from hydration to best foods to eat (including meal plans), to exercise, to food sensitivities, to lab testing. She makes complicated processes understandable. I love the simplicity of her food recommendations and the recap at the end."

—Katherine Erlich, MD, author of *Super Nutrition for Babies*

The Supercharged Method

**YOUR TRANSFORMATION
FROM FATIGUED TO ENERGIZED**

Stacey Francis, D.C.

Publishing support provided by
Ignite Press
5070 N. Sixth St. #189
Fresno, CA 93710
www.IgnitePress.us

ISBN: 979-8-9860255-0-6
ISBN: 979-8-9860255-1-3 (Hardcover)
ISBN: 979-8-9860255-2-0 (E-book)

For bulk purchase and for booking, contact:

Stacey Francis
info@thesuperchargedmethod.com
thesuperchargedmethod.com

Because of the dynamic nature of the Internet, web addresses or links contained in this book may have been changed since publication and may no longer be valid. The content of this book and all expressed opinions are those of the author and do not reflect the publisher or the publishing team. The author is solely responsible for all content included herein.

The information in this book is not intended to replace the care of, or relationship with, a qualified healthcare professional and is not intended as medical advice. It is intended as a sharing of knowledge and information from the research and experience of Dr. Stacey Francis, TheSuperchargedMethod.com, and the experts who have contributed. This information is to be used with the guidance and supervision of a qualified healthcare professional. This information is for educational purposes only, and no guarantees, promises, representations, or warranties of any kind regarding specific or general benefits have been or will be made by Dr. Stacey Francis, her affiliates, or their officers, principals, representatives, agents, or employees. Dr. Stacey Francis is not responsible for, and shall have no liability for any success or failure, act and/or omissions, the appropriateness of the participant's decisions, or the use of or reliance on this information.

Library of Congress Control Number: 2022904267

Cover design by Swamynathan
Edited by Charlie Wormhoudt
Interior design by Jetlaunch

FIRST EDITION

For my husband Tim
and my sons Benjamin and Noah
who believe in me but also know
to hide the cookies and chips.

Acknowledgments

This book would have been written so much sooner if I had the confidence that I know enough. I am a chronic learner, and just like the misconception that fat is evil that we learned 40 years ago, information changes. I fear I will miss something or not be current. But I also realize I am not doing you any favors by holding back and waiting until I know everything or even more. I have to thank my editorial board, teachers, and the doctors who have come before me and have contributed to this book with the information they have shared so generously online and in person. I would also like to thank the doctor who may have shared this book with you. These doctors are the elite in health-care. They have recognized that our current healthcare system is more of a disease management system and have committed their lives to seeking a better result for you. They acknowledge that they can lead you, but it is you who holds the key to your health in the food choices you make, the behaviors you adopt, and the habits you practice. I want to acknowledge you, the reader and owner of this information. As soon as you read the words they become part of you and the knowledge you can use to optimize your health and the health of those around you. You are the reason I wrote this book, and I humbly thank you.

Table of Contents

Preface

MY STORY

I thought I had a poor memory, was stressed out, and just too busy. My head felt foggy more often than not, and when 3 p.m. hit, I needed a nap. Driving on highways gave me highway hypnosis.

Doctors kept passing the buck and telling me my labs were fine. They offered me antidepressants that I didn't want and didn't need. One day everything changed. Driving home from work, I stopped at a light. I watched a woman and a young girl walk across the intersection in front of me. I thought to myself, *Is my car still moving? Is it stopped?* I stepped on the brake harder just to make sure.

And it occurred to me...I shouldn't be on the road. My brain wasn't working, and no one could tell me why.

MY RECOVERY, DISCOVERY, AND MISSION

I knew I had to look outside the conventional system and figure out if I could be fixed. I spent thousands of dollars on courses of nutrition, biochemistry and blood work. It took me years to gather enough information about food sensitivities, thyroid imbalance, blood sugar, anemias, mold exposure, adrenal dysfunction, heavy-metal toxicity—all factors I suspected were at play—before I figured out how to heal my brain.

Now learning comes easy, I have laser-sharp focus, I'm awake all day, and it's safe for me to be on the road.

The silver lining in learning all this the hard way is I'm now able to assist my patients in living a life of clarity, focus, energy, and peace. And that's what I live for.

Introduction

Are you tired? 45% of Americans are, and those are the ones getting sufficient sleep. Would you like to have energy to spare? The Supercharged Method will eliminate the most common and correctable causes of fatigue. It is easy to follow and you can enjoy your life to its fullest knowing you are on a healthy pathway to the energy you are looking for. In this program there are no stimulants or drugs that will cause other problems down the road. *The Supercharged Method* will address blood sugar imbalances, oxygen transport issues from low iron and B vitamins, thyroid issues, adrenal issues, and inflammation.

When people participate in my nutrition programs they are often looking for the same thing that had you pick up this book. They want energy to function throughout the day, clarity to understand the tasks at hand, and the focus to complete them.

When I ask them to forgo caffeine and alcohol much moaning ensues. "I can't live without coffee." "It's my birthday, you mean I can't have a drink?" "You don't understand, I can't poop without my coffee!" "But I'm going away for a girls weekend. I can't be the only one not drinking!" I've heard it all.

Just like you will do after reading Section One of this book, they all clean out their kitchens and pantries, replace inflammatory and processed foods with healthy whole foods, and remove sugar, caffeine, alcohol, juices, and anything artificial. They prepare menus to keep themselves on track. They know they are going to eat three to four whole meals a day without snacking.

Being off caffeine, alcohol, and sugar can make you feel like a truck hit you. Removing these substances can leave you feeling tired, moody, constipated, and miserable. Just like you will soon learn, these participants in my program needed to increase their water intake and be more mindful of resting and repairing their bodies.

Don't run away yet. I know this doesn't sound like a walk in the park, but once your body is free of the addictions and dependencies of using caffeine, alcohol, and sugar and you are providing your body with much needed nutrients, you will be astonished by how much better you feel.

Once the participants break free from the substances that bind them they see the light. They feel better, experience more energy, sleep more soundly, and notice they don't have the cravings they once did. Many notice these changes in a very short time.

This program you are about to embark on is a journey with food and without food. You will eat the foods that serve your body. You will forgo the ones that don't, even if you try to convince me otherwise. Especially if you try to convince me otherwise.

My patients are amazed with the results and by the end of this program I hope you are too.

They often go from this...

"I am on the struggle bus today. One of the reasons is I look forward to Friday and Saturday night dinner all week because we get carry-out on these nights. Obviously not happening today or tomorrow unless Dr. Stacey says I can have something from this place that I have been wanting to try."

To:

"I have to say a huge thank you to Dr. Stacey. I woke up this morning feeling FANTASTIC! I have not felt this good in years. Honestly, probably not in 13 years. Thank you. Whatever seems to be happening, despite my whining, it's working."

—Liz Tkacz Breitner

How often have you hit a brick wall when trying to resolve your lack of energy, clarity, and focus? Was it when you tried the latest fad diet? Was it when you started drinking energy drinks or coffee multiple times a day? I have the hammer to your brick wall. Let's disassemble it together so you can have the energy you need, think clearer than ever, and focus solely on the tasks at hand. ***The Supercharged Method* is a step-by-step guide that will help you hydrate well, sleep great, eat delicious food, and learn to read your labs to achieve optimal—not adequate—wellness.**

Start with whatever steps here float your boat, motivate you, or inspire you and then add another, and another. Soon you will go from Wendy's chicken nuggets and fries, to chili and fries, to chili and a baked potato, to making the chili and baked potato at home and freezing it in portions to eat only half the potato, to adding some vegetables, and so on as you get closer to owning your health and what makes you feel good. If you are inspired to feel amazing in a short period of time, follow these steps to the T. Keep at it and keep putting your health first. Don't give up.

Before You Get Started

"If you do not change direction, you might end up where you are heading."

—Lao Tzu

WHAT IS The Supercharged Method?
The Supercharged Method is five simple steps to gain energy, clarity, and focus.

- Step 1: Prepare your home by removing energy-robbing and inflammatory foods and restocking your kitchen with energy-boosting and anti-inflammatory foods.
- Step 2: Drink half your body weight in ounces of water daily.
- Step 3: Get seven to nine hours of good sleep each night.
- Step 4: Eat one serving of protein and two servings of non-starchy vegetables every three to four hours in a 12-hour-or-less time frame.
- Step 5: Set aside 20 minutes a day to relax and breathe.

The Supercharged Method is five simple steps to gain energy, clarity, and focus. This book breaks down each step and provides tips on how to achieve each one.

WHO THIS BOOK IS FOR...

So you've read the cover and said to yourself, "Yes I am sleepy when I shouldn't be, and yes I do want to be supercharged." Then you wonder, *Is this the right program for me?* You think to yourself, *I've tried other things, how do I know this is different, safe, and effective?*

If you don't know where your fatigue and brain fog are coming from, this book is for you. If you do know, the methods in this book can still help.

If you have never looked at your own blood work this will be a great start. I'm going to make it easy to understand why blood work is important and how to assess the markers. You will learn how to evaluate your health and be an advocate for yourself. You will learn a great deal while reading this book. You may even go out into the world and help your family, friends, and community advocate for their health too.

If you are overly busy this is the perfect book for you. This is a structured system that you can put into your schedule, and I will help make sure you have exactly what you need to do The Supercharged Method well and get the results you are looking for.

If you think you don't have access to blood work because you live in a cave in the remotest part of Timbuktu, this book is still for you. You can follow the steps without getting any labs and still find energy, focus, and clarity.

If you tried another program that made sense to you but didn't work, did you give it enough time? If the answer is no, go back and try it again. It made sense to you. Try again for a longer amount of time and do it by the book. If you have done that and you still don't have the energy, clarity, and focus you are looking for, then it might be a good time to start The Supercharged Method.

If you only have access to processed fast food, then this book is still for you. You can find the healthiest choices at fast food restaurants, and there's a chapter exactly for those situations. But...let me emphasize that you will be removing processed foods in The Supercharged Method, and the difference you will find in your energy, clarity, focus and immunity will blow your socks off.

If you can't afford to buy organic, free-range, and wild-caught food this book is still for you. Although those are the best foods to put into your body, you can still get the results you are looking for from following this method.

If you have a serious disease that is causing your fatigue and brain fog and are working with your doctor on it, run The Supercharged Method by them and ask them to support you on these healthy habits.

If you are vegan, make a concerted effort to include protein-rich foods in your diet when following this method. This may mean including protein shakes, which can be delicious, filling, and satisfying.

If you are on a restricted diet, you can still use this method. You will just need to modify it. You can still follow the basic tenets of the course and regain your energy, focus, and clarity.

If you have hypothyroidism you will learn more about your thyroid and how it works. Since hypothyroidism can also be genetic, The Supercharged Method may even help your children.

Even if you have the best doctors in the world, they can't do this for you. They can guide you, and if they have given you this book they have given you the tools to empower you around your health. They will monitor you to keep you safe, but it's you who needs to do the work to get results.

WHY ARE YOU HERE?

If you are reading this book you likely have not found the answers you are looking for to resolve your fatigue and brain fog, or you are looking to harness all the energy, clarity, and focus you can. No matter why you are here, I'm glad you are. If you take the information in this book and apply it to your lifestyle you will learn how your body works and not only improve your own life but the lives around you. Your spouse, your kids, your family, and your friends will all benefit from you taking charge of your life and teaching them how to transform theirs.

The six most common causes of fatigue and brain fog are:

- Dehydration
- Poor Sleep
- Blood sugar imbalance
- Thyroid dysfunction
- Anemia (including iron deficiency and vitamin B deficiency)
- Adrenal dysfunction
- Inflammation (including autoimmune conditions)

Which causes above could be yours? Are you drinking enough water? Sleeping well enough? Eating in a way that balances your blood sugar? When you improve those areas you may notice you don't need to go any further. If you are still struggling, you can look at your labs which will indicate other "energy robbers" like thyroid imbalance, nutrient deficiencies, and inflammation.

Best case scenario, you get everything you are looking for from adequate water, sleep, and good, balanced food. If you are still struggling after these steps, you can have the blood tests performed. But if you order the lab tests at the beginning, you may have the results by the time you have mastered the first three steps. At that point, you may only need to fine tune your lifestyle.

WHERE ARE YOU NOW?

WORKSHEET ONE: TAKING INVENTORY

Before we can make changes to our lifestyle, we have to evaluate our current behaviors. Below is a worksheet to help you get started. This worksheet is important because we often forget how far we have come and why we want to change our behaviors. Answer the questions honestly and dig deep for answers. Your "why" may change over time, and that is okay. We are all a work in progress.

Write down the foods, drinks, and the quantities you think you will consume during the day and when you think you will be eating and drinking. Throughout the day reflect on how you feel and how your body feels after eating those items. Watch for a pattern. A pattern might look like feeling wired and anxious every time you drink coffee, or waking up at night after eating past 8 p.m. Notice what comes up time and time again. That is the pattern, and if it causes you discomfort, change it.

Here is an example:

Time:	My Plan:	What Actually Happened:
7 a.m.	Wake up and drink 32 oz. water over the next 4 hours	✓ Felt refreshed
10 a.m.	Eat a vegetable omelette and ½ cup berries	✓ Felt alert and satisfied
10:30 a.m.		Drank coffee and felt wired and anxious
11 a.m.	Drink 32 oz. herbal tea over the next 3 hours	Work stress...ate donuts in the conference room instead of journaling my feelings or taking a short walk.
1 p.m.	Eat a large salad with tuna and ½ cup of potatoes	Still stuffed and felt guilty from eating the donuts. Skipped lunch. Felt brain fog and bloated.
2 p.m.	Drink 32 oz. water with electrolytes over the next 2 hours	✓
4 p.m.	Eat hummus, vegetables, and ½ cup of grapes	Work got busy. Didn't take the time to eat.
7 p.m.	Eat chicken, broccoli, spinach, and ½ cup of rice	Felt tired and overly hungry from skipping the last two meals. Ate crackers, chips and ice cream.
9 p.m.	Turn off electronics and wind down	Feeling bloated from over-indulging. Re-commit to following Dr. Stacey's plan tomorrow.

How I feel now	Tired, frustrated, braintired, fed up
Why I think I feel that way	Poor eating habits, work stress, poor planning
How I want to feel	Energized, able to focus more at work, organized
Why I want to feel that way	I want to enjoy my life and have energy to do more fun things like travel

Now it's your turn… (This worksheet and others can be accessed at www.thesuperchargedmethod.com)

Time:	My Plan:	What Actually Happened:

How I feel now	
Why I think I feel that way	
How I want to feel	
Why I want to feel that way	

PREPARE FOR LABS (BLOOD WORK)

This is a good time to get your baseline blood work drawn. Getting a baseline blood work panel will give you some information of what to focus on, but more importantly it will show you how far you have come once you have worked with The Supercharged Method for a few months.

If you are a person who gets yearly blood draws you are ahead of the game. Your doctor is making sure that you will be treated if you develop a disease or disease process. This is good, but it could be great. I call this sick care or disease management if they are checking your blood work yearly and waiting for the values to land outside of the conventional lab range to treat you. These doctors rarely recommend diet improvements or lifestyle changes—not because they don't think they are helpful (although there are those who don't) but because they are waiting for you to request them. At that point, they might guide you, or refer you to a nutritional or lifestyle specialist. That is what I consider "good."

There are also doctors who will acknowledge that there are lab ranges and optimal or functional lab ranges. These are typically narrow ranges that indicate you are functioning at your best and that you are "on point" with your nutrition, sleep, stress, choices, behaviors, habits, and genetic expression. They know if you are between lab range and optimal range there are things you can do to improve your health and prevent disease. This is truly health care, and doctors who take measures to help you prevent disease are "great."

The Supercharged Method is not intended to be used without a health practitioner's oversight. If you are out of lab range, that is the territory that your licensed health practitioner should address. They have spent years evaluating and navigating the intricacies of blood work. Rely on them to help you resolve any values that are out of range.

Directories to find a functional/holistic/integrative doctor near you:

- www.ifm.org
- www.aihm.org
- www.icimed.com
- www.acam.org

The Supercharged Method is specifically, and only, for the ranges that lie between lab range and optimal range. If you order your own blood work and find a test that your doctor doesn't normally run is out of lab range, you need to have them help you bring it back into lab range, but preferably optimal range. You can do The Supercharged Method alongside that treatment.

There are different ways to identify a health problem. Symptoms are one thing, labs are another. Not just any labs. The right labs. Although the labs I'm suggesting are not an extensive list, they are the ones that, when in optimal range, make the most difference with your energy. For a more thorough look at labs, see Section Six.

If you have a health condition, such as anemia, your blood work will show enough abnormality to alert your doctor. An out of lab range would be indicated by an "H" or "L" on your lab report.

The process of your labs moving out of optimal range may be missed if treatment only occurs once you are out of range. You can have symptoms for years (which, in this example, doesn't mean you have anemia, but it could indicate low iron) as you move from optimal health to lower and lower iron levels before the values of your blood work show you are out of range.

We need to look more thoroughly every time blood work is performed, and not just look at whether the levels are in range or not, but how they are moving. Are you barely in range and slowly moving back into a healthy range or more out of range? Let's catch it then, before it's a problem that takes more work to correct.

The following are the labs you can look at to evaluate markers for The Supercharged Method.

You may request these from your doctor or use a lab on your own. They cover blood sugar, anemias, thyroid levels, and inflammation.

Blood Sugar:

- Glucose
- Insulin
- Hemoglobin A1c
- Triglycerides

Anemias:

- Ferritin
- Iron

- Total iron binding capacity
- Mean corpuscular volume
- Mean corpuscular hemoglobin
- Hemoglobin
- Hematocrit
- Methylmalonic acid

Thyroid:

- Thyroid stimulating hormone
- Total thyroxine
- Free thyroxine
- Total triiodothyronine
- Free triiodothyronine
- Reverse triiodothyronine
- Thyroperoxidase antibody
- Thyroglobulin antibody

Inflammation:

- C-reactive protein
- Fibrinogen
- Erythrocyte sedimentation rate
- Homocysteine
- 25 hydroxy vitamin D

THE METHOD

Here is a simple checklist and time table for embarking on The Supercharged Method.

- Week One: Run your baseline blood work.
              Read and implement Section One: Prepare (Clean out and stock up)
- Week Two: Read and implement Section Two: Hydrate (Drink your H20)
- Week Three: Read and implement Section Three: Sleep (Get your 7–9 hours)
- Week Four: Read and implement Section Four: Eat (1+2 Every 3–4 in 12)
- Week Five: Read and implement Section Five: Chill (20 minutes to restore)
- Week Six: Maintain the healthy habits you are establishing as you read through the rest of the sections.

Each week builds upon the previous week. You should still hydrate while getting seven to nine hours of sleep. Eventually you should be practicing all these steps. You will find greater health by developing these steps into consistent habits.

Draw follow-up blood work after maintaining The Supercharged Method for three months. At that point you will have adopted some kick-ass habits, and if there is any blood work that needs to be improved. you will know how to move forward by tightening up your program or consulting with a doctor if needed.

HOW LONG IS THE SUPERCHARGED METHOD?

Some of you will methodically work through The Supercharged Method, no problem. Some of you will get caught up on this or that, get in your own way or get overwhelmed. For those people, I want you to take as long as you need. Figure out what works for you and what doesn't. Start with as many of the foundation steps as you can manage. See how you are feeling. If you are even feeling 10% better, that's great!!! Note that. Know what you did to feel 10% better. Then continue or tweak The Supercharged Method knowing that if it goes south you come back to your 10% program. If it gets better, note that and that becomes your new baseline foundation to return to as you tweak The Supercharged Method. Sometimes you will want to try an off-program food or activity. Note how you feel and know to come back to baseline. Once you are comfortable with the program, be consistent for three months before evaluating your progress and redoing your lab work.

In my clinic I offer The Supercharged Cleanse. It is two weeks off caffeine and alcohol before day one of a strict ten to 21-day program. On day one we start following The Supercharged Method as described in this book with an addition of supplements that help with detoxification and removing some of the highest allergenic foods such as milk, peanuts, wheat, and soy. The experiences of the participants are at the end of this book.

Ask yourself, "What are you willing to do to get the results you desire?"

SECTION ONE

PREPARE

"How can I create an environment that will naturally bring about my desired change?"

—James Clear

CHAPTER 1

THE BEST ENVIRONMENT

My patients come in for a variety of reasons, and most of them, whether they realize it or not, have blood sugar imbalances. The recommendations in this book will first and foremost address these imbalances. Even if this is not your issue, you would benefit from the food and behavior choices in The Supercharged Method. Even sleep is disrupted if your blood sugar is off. When you follow The Supercharged Method you will, at the very least, learn what a balanced blood sugar feels like and how much more energy, clarity, and focus you will have if you keep it balanced.

Blood sugar imbalances often come from foods you thought were "healthy," or hoped that they were. We are not only replacing candy, cookies, cakes, soda and fruit juice—which all contain sugar and barely any nutrients—we are also replacing chips, processed foods, chemical-laden foods, and otherwise inflammatory foods. We are replacing all of the above with whole foods that mother nature made and that have the nutrients your body needs.

Remember that figuring out how to marry your love of sweets, fats, and salt with healthy choices that benefit your health is a lifelong journey. Eating whole, delicious foods that you love and look forward to is the ultimate goal. It can be an uncomfortable process to move away from processed, packaged, addictive foods, but you can do it. Whether you do it because you are scared to lose your eyesight or your toes due to uncontrolled diabetes or you do it to feel powerful and in control as you gain back lost energy, keep modifying and tweaking and working with The Supercharged Method and your support team, and don't give up.

Set up your environment to succeed. If you have junk food lying around and you love junk food, you will inevitably eat it until you have more control over your choices. If you only have delicious healthy choices in your refrigerator and pantry, guess what you are more likely to choose? Set yourself up powerfully. Keep your kitchen stocked with your favorite healthy foods. Know the restaurants that have the healthiest choices. Know how to read an ingredient label. Know what it takes to make your body feel and function at its best. I will teach you all this and more and you will have more energy, clarity, and focus than you could have hoped for.

HOW TO READ INGREDIENTS ON A NUTRITION LABEL

Let's start with: If a food item was made naturally and you can identify it, it's probably a good ingredient. If you don't know what an ingredient is, your body probably doesn't either. The manufacturers of junk food will do their best to hide sugar, artificial colors, flavors and preservatives in their products and may use terms you are not familiar with that might get past you.

Being able to identify whole foods and whole food ingredients is a great skill to have to take control of your health and the health of your family.

THE ORDER LISTED IS IMPORTANT

Ingredients are listed by weight. The first ingredient has the most weight in the product; the second has less weight than the first but more than the third, and so on. As an example let's take "brand name" Simply Granola. The word "Simply" can be deceiving since we may think "Simply" means nothing bad is added. Granola is often thought of as a healthy food, but it typically has a lot of sugar in its ingredients. The first ingredients in our example are whole grain rolled oats, then whole grain rolled wheat, then brown sugar. The sugar is listed before any nuts so there is more brown sugar per weight than pecans which is after canola oil (an unhealthy oil), inulin (a fiber) and whey (a milk protein). If we keep reading down the ingredient list we would find another form of sugar (honey) and another unhealthy oil (sunflower oil). Definitely not a "health" food.

I'm sorry for picking on granola if you are a granola fan. Try a trail mix instead, made of a variety of nuts and seeds (that you can toast lightly) and freeze-dried berries.

NOTE THE SERVING SIZE AND SERVINGS PER PACKAGE

When I was a kid there was nothing better than waking up on a Saturday morning to eat my favorite sugary cereal while watching cartoons. I first started paying attention to nutrition labels in chiropractic school. Before I was knowledgeable about nutrition and how it affected the body, breakfast cereal was still a staple in my diet. One serving of cereal barely filled half my bowl, and I was still hungry after eating it.

A serving size is a standardized amount of food. It is noted on the nutrition label of most foods or can be found online. A portion size can be larger or smaller than the serving size. Some cans of tuna will show that the contents of one can is one serving, but you might split that into two portions. You will be getting either ten grams or 20 grams of protein depending on what portion size you choose. Choose a portion size based on what nutrients you want to consume. In a meal plan I might suggest a serving of hummus. A serving of hummus is often considered two tablespoons and contains only two grams of protein. You may choose to increase that portion to a quarter cup to increase your protein for that meal or, knowing that you are only getting two grams of protein, have more protein in another meal that day.

I learned to pay attention to the serving size and how many servings are in the package in order to make good choices when planning meals. You need to know that sugar, salt, and fat are poured into processed food to make them addictive and delicious. The manufacturers create the perfect balance to overstimulate your brain to make you want more.

If we go back to my cereal example, you can now see why that magical combination of sugar, salt, and fat (and bright colors) were so appealing but can leave you feeling empty.

STOCK UP ON WHAT YOU LIKE AND WHAT YOU EAT (BUT ALSO TRY NEW THINGS)

I am obsessed with watching meal prep videos. I just love how the meals are organized and accessible. It is picture perfect, literally. If you have a desire to do that I applaud you. If, on the other hand, you are like me and are winning if you have cleaned out the refrigerator just enough to cram in a variety of healthy food choices in every nook and cranny, you also rock.

Having a variety of proteins, vegetables, healthy fats and other complex carbohydrates makes it convenient, easy, and, dare I say, fun to create amazing meals that will fit in The Supercharged Method.

PROTEINS

Pick proteins that are as natural as possible with as few ingredients as possible and not modified to improve taste or extend shelf life. Avoid proteins that have a list of ingredients as long as a drugstore receipt. Hotdogs and bologna are examples of proteins to avoid. These processed protein sources contain chemicals and preservatives that can contribute to disease. Organic grass-fed dairy, beef, and poultry, humanely treated, are the best animal proteins to purchase, but they can be cost prohibitive at times. If eating healthy protein is important to you, you can make these protein sources go farther by mixing them into soups and stews with beans or lentils.

Choose organic and grass-fed:

- Beef
- Bison
- Chicken
- Pork
- Lamb

- Venison
- Turkey
- Quail
- Duck
- Game meat

Wild-caught:

- Alaskan salmon
- Mackerel
- Anchovies
- Sardines
- Herring
- Cod
- Mahi-mahi
- Perch
- Rainbow trout
- Barramundi
- Striped bass

- Char
- Alaskan pollock
- Skipjack tuna
- Squid
- Snails
- Clams
- Oysters
- Crab
- Lobster
- Scallops

Avoid the following fish due to risk of increased toxins and heavy metals:

- Tilapia
- Tilefish
- Swordfish

- Shark
- King mackerel

Choose organic and rBGH-free (recombinant Bovine Growth Hormone):

- Eggs
- Milk
- Yogurt
- Cheese

My younger son, Noah, reminded me recently of one of his memories growing up. On our quest to better health, I came across a dilemma. Noah was a picky eater and he had a fondness for milk. Aside from breast milk I don't think milk is the best food for weaned humans but at the time I was desperate to feed him anything. The beneficial enzymes and probiotics in raw milk versus commercial milk had me searching for a source. I had some patients inform me that I could purchase a share of a cow and have access to the raw milk it provided. Noah recalls the long drive to meet our cow and the one jug of milk we enjoyed before we decided that driving an hour for milk did not fit our family plan. I'm happy to say that since then he has welcomed more variety into his meals.

Nuts are often considered a protein but are a much better fat source. If you are vegetarian I recommend getting protein wherever you can, which is why you will see nuts and seeds here. If you are not a vegetarian, use one tablespoon of nuts, seeds, or nut/seed butter as a fat source or a supplemental protein source and not a main protein source.

Choose organic:

- Almonds
- Pine nuts
- Walnuts
- Macadamia nuts

- Hazelnuts
- Cashews
- Pumpkin seeds
- Sesame seeds
- Chia seeds
- Hemp seeds (also called hemp hearts)
- Sunflower seeds
- Nut or seed butters

Beans and legumes are sources of protein and carbohydrates. Once again, if you are a vegetarian you will use it as a protein source. If you are not a vegetarian, use a serving as a carbohydrate source or a supplemental protein source combined with a fish or animal source. An example would be beef and bean soup.

Choose organic:

- Beans
- Lentils
- Chickpeas
- Split peas
- Edamame
- Tofu

Protein powders are convenient and can provide protein for vegetarians and those who prefer to drink their meals. Be mindful of the ingredient list. Avoid artificial sweeteners, colors, flavors and preservatives. Choose a protein powder with preferably 15–20 grams of protein. It is best to find a "single ingredient" protein powder and add your own fruit and healthy natural sweetener. Look for the ones that have organic egg, bone broth, pea/rice, or whey (unless you are sensitive to dairy).

Most protein bars are really more like candy bars. They are not recommended due to their low amount of protein, high carbohydrate count, high calorie count, and less than optimal ingredients. Jerky and other animal protein bars are the only exception since the main ingredient is animal protein and few other ingredients. Choose grass-fed, antibiotic-free, and humanely-treated or wild-caught sources. Examples are:

- EPIC bars
- Chomps sticks
- Wild Zora bars
- DNX bars
- Nick's Sticks
- Thrive Market
- Country Archer
- Lorissa's
- PaleoValley
- Grass Run Farms
- Caveman Foods
- Mission Meats

Avoid Tilapia

Tilapia is a common farm-raised whitefish of many species. It is sourced predominantly out of China with questionable farming and safety practices. Although wild-caught tilapia would be acceptable, it is hard to find. Tilapia is also higher in omega-6 oils than anti-inflammatory omega-3 oils. Americans tend to have a diet higher in omega-6 oils from a higher consumption of vegetable oils. This added omega-6 source can tip the scales into an inflammatory state. A March 2016 article in the journal *Nutrients* shows an increase in the omega-6 to omega-3 fatty acid ratio increases the risk for obesity which is an inflammatory condition.

Avoid Tilefish, Swordfish, Shark, and King Mackerel

These fish often contain dangerous levels of mercury which is harmful to our brain cells and can cause heart disease, memory problems, difficulty focusing, and nervous system damage.

These, like other large fish, such as Chilean sea bass, grouper, and larger tuna like albacore, for example, live longer and eat the smaller fish ending up with more toxins. Remember when eating tuna to choose the wild-caught skipjack variety.

Seed

Hemp seed is one of my favorite vegetarian proteins. It is a complete protein which means it has all the essential amino acids that the body cannot make and has to get from food. It is easy to use, widely available and the taste is neutral and can be turned into either a sweet or savory dish. Three tablespoons gives you just under ten grams of protein, 2.6 grams of carbohydrate, 1.2 grams of fiber, 15 grams of fat and 166 calories. In the meal plan section you will see how hemp seeds can be used to make hot cereal, cold cereal, and bump up the protein in shakes and smoothies. You can also use hemp seed in vegetable stir fries and salads to get your protein fix. It is a source of omega fatty acids, vitamin E, iron, magnesium, and zinc. Hemp oil contains both omega-6 and omega-3 oils. Most omega-6 oils from vegetable oils are inflammatory and I suggest you avoid them. Hemp seed, however, contains Gamma-Linoleic Acid or GLA. Even though it is an omega-6 oil it is an anti-inflammatory oil and studies suggest that it may even protect DNA. Hemp seeds are a good choice for a vegetarian protein source.

VEGETABLES

Avoid canned food. When I was growing up, a popular meal was tomato soup and grilled cheese. Back then, the tomato soup had a tinny taste from the acidic tomatoes pulling the metal from the can into the soup. Many cans are still made with aluminum that can leach into the food that it contains. Over time the canning industry started lining their cans with a plastic called bisphenol A or BPA. BPA was discovered to be a carcinogen and endocrine disruptor, which means that it may cause cancer and glandular dysfunction. An October 2015 article in the journal *Reproductive Toxicology* reports that BPA targets breast tissue. BPA was detected in 7% of fresh and frozen foods, and a whopping 73% of canned foods. Don't mess with the ladies, avoid vegetables in cans. Choose fresh and frozen vegetables.

Whenever possible, choose organic vegetables in their naturally harvested season. Also opt for non-starchy or low glycemic vegetables. The glycemic index is a system that ranks food based on how the food impacts blood-sugar levels. (Read more about it in the chapter Eating to Balance Blood Sugar.)

Choose from the following low-glycemic vegetables:

Artichokes	Cauliflower	Greens
Arugula	Celery	Green beans
Asparagus	Chard	Herbs
Bok choy	Collard greens	Jicama
Broccoli	Cucumber	Kale
Broccoli rabe	Eggplant	Leeks
Brussels sprouts	Endive	Lettuce
Cabbage	Garlic	Mushrooms

Okra

Onions

Pea shoots

Peppers

Purslane

Radishes

Rutabaga

Scallions

Shallots

Spinach

Sprouts

Sugar snap/
Snow peas

Summer squash

Tomatoes

Turnips

Try to include foods from these categories of vegetables each day:

- Anti-inflammatory and cell protective cruciferous and sulfur containing vegetables: Onions, mushrooms, cabbage, broccoli, cauliflower, Brussels sprouts, asparagus, shallot, leeks and garlic
- Gut healthy pre- and probiotic vegetables: fermented vegetables, sauerkraut, kimchi, pickles
- Nutrient-rich dark leafy greens: Arugula, kale, spinach, swiss chard, collard greens, bok choy, mustard greens, dandelion greens, turnip greens, beet greens, watercress, broccoli rabe
- Iodine-rich seaweed and sea vegetables: kelp, dulse, kombu, nori, wakame, arame, spirulina, chlorella

Limit these higher glycemic vegetables to a half cup per serving:

Beets

Carrots

Corn

Parsnip

Potatoes (Sweet and White)

Split peas/
Garden peas

Yams

When I was working with my mentor and cousin, Rob Radtke, he would have this stinky jar of sour milk on the kitchen counter in the clinic. It was my job to dole it out to patients and to top it off with more milk when it was running low. I miss the way he laughingly tormented me with that stinky concoction. Of the many things he taught me, the importance of a healthy gut biome was one of them. That stinky jar of milk was full of probiotics that soothed the bellies of many patients. The benefits of probiotics are now well known. Whether you get them from fermented vegetables or cultured milk, probiotics are an important nutrient to have in your diet.

FRUIT

Choose fresh and avoid canned or fruit in syrup. Fruit is legitimately called nature's candy. It is easy to overindulge in the sweet stuff so limit fruit to half cup servings.

Apples	Lime	Pears
Apricots	Mandarins	Persimmon
Bananas	Mangos	Plums
Blueberries	Nectarines	Raspberries
Grapefruit	Orange	Strawberries
Honeydew	Papaya	Watermelon
Kiwi	Passionfruit	Blackberries
Lemons	Peaches	

There is an annual list that identifies the fruits and vegetables that are recommended to buy organic due to high levels of pesticides. It is called the Dirty Dozen, and you can find it through the Environmental Working Group at www.EWG.org.

OILS AND FATS

Every cell of your body is made of fat. Cells have a phospholipid membrane which means your cells are both water soluble and fat soluble. The fat soluble vitamins are vitamins A, D, E, and K, and they need to be taken with fat to be absorbed. That is why you will often see these as supplements in a gel cap suspended in an oil.

Oils are liquid at room temperature, and fats are solid at room temperature. For our purposes here, I will refer to all fats and oils interchangeably. There are a few things to consider when choosing a fat to use for cooking. One, is it a healthy fat, and two, is it the right healthy fat?

Healthy cooking oils include olive oil, avocado oil, coconut oil, lard, butter, and ghee. Ghee is butter that has had its lactose or milk sugar removed. This is also called clarified butter. These healthy oils should be cold pressed, purchased and stored in dark glass bottles. Light degrades these oils instantly so it's important to keep the lid on when not in use. Store them in a cool area, not next to the stove unless you can use it up within a couple weeks.

Fats such as trans fats, hydrogenated oil, canola oil, soybean oil, vegetable oil, corn oil, cottonseed oil, sunflower oil, safflower oil, margarine, shortening, and peanut oil contribute to inflammation in the body and are therefore considered dangerous fats. The most commonly used oil in processed food is canola oil. Canola oil is cheap and often genetically modified. It is heated and then treated with a chemical solvent called hexane to extract the oil and heated again at a high temperature to remove the hexane.

These fats are high in omega-6. When you eat too many omega-6 oils, relative to omega-3 oils, you may find yourself dealing with water retention which can lead to high blood pressure. You may also be more susceptible to blood clots that can lead to a heart attack or stroke, as shown in a May 2019 research article in the publication *Open Heart*. Dementia and Alzheimer's disease have also been linked to consumption of these dangerous oils.

Grapeseed Oil

Grapeseed oil is also an omega-6 oil. It has a high smoke point at 420 degrees fahrenheit. Some people use it in cooking as an olive oil alternative because of its high smoke point and mild flavor, but like the other omega-6 oils, when there is an abundance, and not enough omega-3 oils, inflammation can occur. Even worse, omega-6 oils can decrease the metabolism of healthy plant-based omega oils like flax and walnut to the important EPA and DHA compounds that are anti-inflammatory and brain protective by almost 50%.

All fats and oils heated past their smoke point become dangerous to the human body. Heating an oil past its smoke point or reheating an oil at high temperatures can create carcinogenic free radicals which are cancer causing compounds, as noted in an August 2016 article in the journal *Toxicology Reports*. The bottom line: Don't heat oil past its smoke point.

Smoke Point Chart for Healthy Oils and Fats

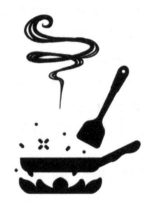

	FAHRENHEIT	CELCIUS
BUTTER	200-250	120-150
EXTRA VIRGIN COCONUT OIL	350	177
LARD	370	188
EXTRA VIRGIN OLIVE OIL	375	191
AVOCADO OIL	375-400	190-205
GHEE OR CLARIFIED BUTTER	450	230

Healthy Cooking Oils

- Avocado
- Coconut
- Olive
- Ghee
- Butter
- Lard

CARB-IER CARBS

Grains

Grains are seeds from plants. If the plants are grass-like then the seeds can be made into a cereal. Examples of grains that create cereals are corn, wheat, and rice. If the plants are not grass-like the meal that they make are called pseudo-cereals. Examples of pseudo-cereals are buckwheat, amaranth, and quinoa.

Whole grains have three parts. The hard, outer shell that contains fiber, minerals, and antioxidants called the bran. A middle layer called the endosperm which is mostly made up of carbs. And the inner germ layer that contains vitamins, minerals, and protein. Where whole grain contains all three parts, refined grains only contain the carb-heavy endosperm. Even with some vitamins and minerals added back in making them "fortified" they can't compete with the nutritional value of whole grains.

- Amaranth
- Barley
- Brown rice
- Buckwheat
- Corn
- Flaxseed
- Millet
- Rice
- Rye
- Whole Wheat

Wheat berries

We hear it so often that "choose organic" mostly falls on deaf ears but there are reasons it is important to choose organic. I could write a whole book on the chemicals that are found in our food supply but I will keep it to this one statistic. According to the Environmental Working Group's analysis of data from the federal Department of Agriculture, nearly 70% of non-organic fresh produce sold in the United States contains residues of potentially harmful chemical pesticides. That was a disturbing statistic for me to find because when I started teaching this information 20 years ago the figure was 35% and I thought that was high.

Now that you understand the importance of organic, there is a resource that provides the most heavily laden pesticide crops and the foods that you can safely buy without being organic. The Environmental Working Group website www.ewg.org provides a yearly dirty dozen list that are the foods you want to buy organic and a clean fifteen list that you may choose to buy non-organic.

Gluten

Gluten is a protein found in wheat and other grains (wheat, rye, barley, spelt and sometimes oats). Many people are sensitive to gluten and do not realize it. The digestive enzymes that our body uses to break down food also break down gluten, specifically an enzyme called protease. But protease cannot break down gluten completely. When undigested gluten or other food make their way to the small intestine it can cause an immune response that makes that food less tolerated in the future. It can go as far as creating an autoimmune disease such as celiac or non-celiac gluten sensitivity.

Dr. William Davis, author of *Wheat Belly*, has a lot to say about why we all should avoid gluten. He shares that the protein in wheat and other grains are poorly digested in human bodies as opposed to the proteins in animal protein like eggs, fish, and beef. The compounds that remain are called peptides. Peptides from gluten protein stimulate opioid receptors in the brain. This stimulates appetite and makes you want more of it.

Complex carbohydrates are touted as beneficial from the American Heart Association, American Diabetes Association, and other well-known establishments. The complex carbohydrate of wheat and grain is called Amylopectin A. Amylopectin A is broken down immediately in the mouth as the enzyme amylase in saliva converts it into sugar. This can contribute to blood sugar imbalance which is another reason to avoid gluten and even grains like barley and oats.

Gluten can cause brain fog, fatigue, skin rashes, auto-immunity, and gastrointestinal issues. You may not have any symptoms but find you have high inflammatory markers in your blood work that gluten can contribute to. Avoiding gluten products can ensure that you are not contributing to this sensitivity. A trial of going completely gluten free (not one iota) may reveal a sensitivity that you didn't even know you had. I suggest you give it a try.

SAUCES, SPICES AND HERBS

Herbs and spices are typically safe to eat and provide a multitude of health benefits in addition to creating a variety of flavors. These can be sprayed heavily with pesticides so choose organic when possible and mind any allergies.

When purchasing salt, which is a necessary mineral in addition to a flavor enhancer, purchase sea salt. Avoid refined table salt. Refined salt has had the minerals removed, usually with a chemical process that leaves in dangerous toxins. Sea salt is the best choice because it provides important minerals and is free of the chemical toxins. If you notice that you are more bloated, retain water, or have more headaches, you may be getting too much refined salt.

Sauces are best homemade. The food industry loves putting sugar and vegetable oils into sauces and dressings. Primal Kitchen is one of a select few brands that is mindful of their ingredients. Make sure to read the labels if you do buy sauces on a shelf.

SWEETENERS

Years ago we didn't realize the impact sugar has on the brain, blood vessels, thyroid, pancreas...I could go on. We know a great deal more now, and when we look at the amount of sugar in a product, we need to consider the serving size and if that is the actual serving size that will be eaten. One 12 ounce can of Coke has 39 grams of sugar. The American Heart Association recommends no more than 36 grams of sugar in a day and the Scientific Advisory Committee on Nutrition recommends no more than 25 grams of sugar per day if you are wanting to avoid diabetes. Two Oreo cookies contain 21 grams of sugar. How many people do you know who only eat two Oreos at a sitting? The five Oreos you actually eat surpasses even the AHA recommendations.

Look for products that do not have sugar in the first five ingredients, and make sure the number of grams of sugar per serving is well under ten. It is easy to eat more than one serving when sugar is involved.

Here are common forms of the many hidden names of sugar:

Anything with the word "syrup," or "sugar," or ending with "-ose"

Agave

Barley malt

Beet sugar

Brown sugar

Cane juice

Caramel

Caster sugar

Coconut palm sugar

Coconut sugar

Confectioner's sugar

Corn sweetener

Corn syrup

Crystalline fructose

D-ribose

Date sugar

Dehydrated cane sugar

Dextrin

Dextrose

Ethyl maltol

Fructose

Fruit juice

Galactose

Glucose

Golden sugar

Grape sugar	Molasses
High fructose corn syrup	Muscovado
Honey	Nectar
Isoglucose	Palm sugar
Lactose	Rice syrup
Malt	Saccharose
Maltodextrin	Sorghum syrup
Maltose	Treacle
Mannose	Turbinado sugar
Maple syrup	

We are programmed to like sweet things. When we are exposed to them daily, it is hard to say no. Despite our decades-long obsession with diets and "what to eat," obesity, diabetes and heart disease are on the rise. As our stress levels increase with politics, pandemics and the daily struggles of jobs, kids, and relationships, it becomes harder to not "bliss out" on the dopamine rush of sugar in the form of cakes, cookies, candies, bread, and alcohol.

Dopamine is our "want what we don't have" chemical. It is produced in the brain and gives us desire. Desire to get out of bed, desire to feed ourselves, and desire to socialize. It travels along the reward pathway in our brain resulting in a feeling of bliss, happiness, and anticipation. Eating increases dopamine which is why it is so easy to overeat when you are stressed out or feeling down. Be aware of this so you can choose a healthier form of stress relief. Things that cause an overproduction of dopamine are illicit drugs, sex, alcohol, video gaming, social media scrolling, flour, and sugar. Although both carbohydrates, a piece of fruit releases more dopamine than broccoli because of the sugar content. Concentrated fruit such as fruit juice releases even more dopamine and straight sugar releases more than juice. This is why there is no juicing on The Supercharged Method. Dopamine release is a wonderful feeling and important for motivation but it's also easy to lose control.

The following list is natural sugars, but they *do* spike insulin levels and should be avoided. Choosing to abstain from sweets with the exception of whole fruit is recommended.

Avoid:

- Honey
- Maple syrup
- Molasses
- Rice syrup
- Coconut sugar

Sugar-Free Sweeteners

Luckily, there are substitutes for sugar and artificial sweeteners that are safe to use as long as they agree with your digestive tract and don't give you gas, bloating, diarrhea, or stomach cramps. They typically do not contain calories since they are not absorbed in the intestinal tract and are derived from food sources. They have minimal effect on insulin, causing them to be low on the glycemic index and safe for those who want to balance their blood sugar. In fact xylitol, although dangerous to dogs, can fight ear infections, help remineralize enamel on your teeth and can help you absorb B vitamins and calcium.

If you cannot control your sweet tooth or just feel something sweet "completes you," the following list of sugar-free sweeteners will not spike blood sugar. Some are many times sweeter than sugar, and a small amount can go far. One of my favorite authors is nutritionist Maria Emmerich. She promotes a ketogenic diet, but even if you are not following a ketogenic diet, you will love her recipes. She is a food magician when it comes to turning your favorite sugar-laden dessert into a sugar-free, naturally sweetened, protein-rich, culinary delight.

Acceptable natural sweeteners:

- Stevia
- Monk fruit
- Sugar alcohols (erythritol, xylitol, maltitol)
- Allulose
- Katemfe Fruit/Thaumatin

Avoid: Acesulfame, aspartame, sucralose, and saccharin.

In an August, 2021 study in *Nutritional Neuroscience*, they found that although erythritol and xylitol did not increase insulin and glucose levels like glucose does, these two natural sweeteners did increase satiety. This is good news. It means that these natural sweeteners can supply you with the feeling of satisfaction without the fat storage and blood sugar spikes that glucose produces.

I'm able to help my patients balance their blood sugar more effectively because I work to balance mine as well. I am sensitive to imbalance and can share with my patients the foods that affect me.

For example, I'm always checking out the latest protein bars. Although choosing to eat whole foods is wiser, we all have busy lives and I'd much rather chow down on a high-protein, low-carb, no-artificial-sweetener bar than ignore my hunger cues and end up eating my face off. One day I discovered a new bar, and it looked delicious, but after eating that protein bar, I felt like someone gave me my blankie, my favorite stuffed animal, and shut off the lights. I fell asleep where I stood. Now I warn my patients to test out everything they eat so they know what zaps their energy too.

CONVENIENT FOODS

I'm all for convenience. If you're always on the go, you can still plan for healthy snacks and ways to add protein in your diet.

- Keep snack-size fruit and vegetable portions easily accessible in your fridge or on the countertop.
- Add fruit and vegetables to salads.
- Add proteins and vegetables to stir-fries, soups, and stews.
- Add fruit, vegetables, and proteins to smoothies. Adding avocado, riced cauliflower, and spinach to smoothies is barely detectable in fruit or cocoa powder-flavored smoothies.

- Keep non-perishable food in the car or at work, like 100% grass-fed beef or turkey sticks or jerky, seaweed snack packs, kale chips, protein bars, apples, packets of nuts and seeds, packs of nut butters, freeze-dried fruit, and cans of wild-caught fish.

BETTER/BEST LIST

If you are ready to dive right in, the following list shows the best choices of food and drink for the quickest route to blood sugar balancing, nutrient intake, and inflammation reduction. If you need more of a transition from the standard American diet to a better diet, that is shown as well. Don't beat yourself up, do the best you can, and if you have a situation that causes your food choices to go to "hell-in-a-handbasket," give yourself some grace and come back to The Supercharged Method as soon as you can.

Remove	Better Alternative	Best Choice
Soda	Stevia / monk fruit-sweetened, no-artificial-color soda	Water
Juice	Fresh squeezed juice with pulp	Water infused with fruit
Candy	Stevia / monk fruit-sweetened, no-artificial-color candy, figs, raisins, or dates	Fresh fruit
Chips	Homemade using healthy oils and flours	Crunchy vegetables, nuts, olives

Remove	Better Alternative	Best Choice
Cookies	Cookies that are banana or date sweetened with healthy oils and flours	Fresh fruit
Crackers	Homemade using healthy oils and flours	Crunchy vegetables
Ice Cream	Homemade using pureed fruit	Pureed frozen fruit
Salad dressings	Whole ingredients and healthy oils	Homemade with healthy oils
Sauces	Whole ingredients and healthy oils	Homemade with healthy oils
Condiments	Whole ingredients and healthy oils	Homemade with healthy oils
Dips	Hummus, guacamole, and pesto	Homemade
Milk chocolate	Dark chocolate	Stevia / monk fruit-sweetened dark chocolate
Pro-cessed meat	Reputable processed meat like Apple-gate Farms	Grass-fed meat, locally sourced
Skim milk	Organic whole milk	Hemp milk (if dairy sensitive)
Commer-cial bread	Homemade bread with sprouted whole grains	Lettuce wraps or slices of sweet potato
Commer-cial eggs	Organic, free-range eggs	Chia or flaxseed for binding in recipes (if egg sensitive)
Canola or vegetable oils	Avocado oil, olive oil, coconut oil, ghee, or butter	Organic versions of Avo-cado oil, olive oil, coconut oil, ghee, or butter
Mixed nuts	Nuts with sea salt and without added oils or sugar	Unroasted and sea salted nuts

CHAPTER HIGHLIGHTS

★ Empty your refrigerator and pantry of any products with sugar and inflammatory oils.

★ Pay attention to serving size.

★ Avoid processed foods that are created to be addictive.

★ Fill your kitchen with healthy protein sources, fresh or frozen organic vegetables, healthy fats, healthy carbohydrates, clean sauces, herbs, spices, and sea salt.

★ Choose organic, grass-fed, grass-finished, and wild-caught whenever possible.

Chapter 2

FOOD INDUSTRY SECRETS

I remember when I was a kid, my mom brought home these delightful fat-free chocolate cake-like cookies that looked like little pillows with a thin layer of white filling covered in a layer of chocolate. My mom was health conscious and, like the rest of the world, falsely believed that fat was the enemy. I remember our joy of discovering and eating these "fat-free" biscuits of deliciousness. Proud of our health awareness, we sought out all the delectable "fat-free" foods not realizing that the high sugar content and processed carbohydrates inched us closer and closer to a state of disease. I developed an autoimmune thyroid disease and both my mother and father suffered from the effects of diabetes and heart disease. All of which could have been avoided if we would have known better and done better.

It has become so common to be diagnosed with diabetes and heart disease that it is almost a rite of passage in the United States and other developed countries. About one in ten people in the United States have diabetes. And 90–95% of them have Type 2 Diabetes. A January 2019 report published in the AHA journal *Circulation* said an astonishing 48% of adults in the United States have cardiovascular disease. And autoimmune diseases are racing to catch up, increasing by 50% over the last 25 years. The tragic reality is that many are still convinced that fat is the enemy and not sugar, processed carbs, vegetable oils, artificial colors, preservatives, and...ok, trans fats. Often when processed food companies remove fat from a product, they replace it with three times as much refined flour and sugar.

The struggle is real, and I am not immune to it. Tonight I came home from a long day at work after only a few hours of sleep due to daylight savings time and writing too long past my bedtime. I talked to myself in the car, telling myself that I should take a 20-minute nap as soon as I get home. Once home, our dog needed to be fed, a friend called and wanted to talk, and my family was hungry. No nap. I soon found myself grazing on cheese, chocolate, and nuts. When my son brought home fried plantains from our favorite Cuban restaurant and my husband brought home Ben and Jerry's, I didn't have one brain cell left to remember how horrible I'd feel after eating fried food and ice cream. I can't blame that entirely on the food industry, but it sure knows the magic formula to make us want to indulge.

AN ADDICTIVE COMBINATION

The food industry makes packaged and processed food incredibly desirable with just the right ratios of sugar, fat, and salt. So desirable that we have an epidemic of obesity, heart disease, and Type 2 diabetes. The right combination of these ingredients gives us a feeling of being gratified, satisfied, joyful, and comfortable. There is even a term for it, coined by market researcher and psychophysicist, Howard Moskowitz. It is called the "bliss point." Once the food industry added a crunchy component, it was game over. The public not only desired these "foods," it craved them. And who was specifically targeted and vulnerable? Kids. Even though adults may be able to moderate their consumption better than children, the combination of sugar, fat, and salt is so desirable because it actually causes an increase in dopamine production in the brain, making processed snacks and treats addictive to all age groups. To make a bad situation worse, some people have a genetic variation that makes them especially vulnerable to the effects of processed foods on their brain.

THE MOST EVIL OF SUGARS

There is nothing cheaper, sweeter, or more quickly absorbed into the body than high fructose corn syrup, also called corn syrup or corn sugar. You will find it in commercially made soda, cereals, cookies, and cakes, but it can also be hiding in food products that are not necessarily that sweet like dressings and bread. That is why it's important to read labels.

Fruit has fructose, but it also has fiber, vitamins, minerals, and enzymes that help with its metabolism and absorption. High fructose corn syrup has no nutritive value.

According to a December 2017 article published in *PLoS* (Public Library of Science) *One*, high fructose corn syrup can induce metabolic dysregulation. Metabolic dysregulation is when your body reacts to certain factors like high blood sugar, high blood pressure, high triglycerides in the blood, and excess belly fat. These factors can increase your risk of heart disease, stroke, and Type 2 diabetes.

Glucose is fuel that the body uses for energy. Excess glucose can be stored in the liver to be used later. Fructose is quickly broken down (metabolized) in the liver. Excess fructose increases your triglycerides and leads to non-alcoholic fatty liver disease. Fructose overconsumption also increases risk of heart attack, stroke, obesity, and diabetes. It can even lead to gout in some individuals.

Functional medicine expert Dr. Mark Hymen explains that fructose goes straight to the liver and produces fat by triggering the buildup of triglycerides and cholesterol. Fructose can then create tears in the lining of the blood vessels and tears in the intestinal lining which allows toxins, bigger food particles, and bacteria to get into the bloodstream, causing inflammation and food sensitivities.

ARTIFICIAL SWEETENERS

Aspartame (Equal), sucralose (Splenda), saccharin (Sweet-n-Low) and acesulfame k are all chemical look-alikes of sugar and are linked to the one thing people consume them for: weight control. Not only do these artificial sweeteners contribute to weight GAIN, but they are also linked to diabetes, kidney disease, and metabolic dysfunction, which can cause fatigue. It's just another reason why you may be tired.

ARTIFICIAL COLORS

A seven-year-old patient was referred to me because he couldn't focus at school and was frequently being sent to the principal's office for behavioral problems. When he came into my office he was super chatty and quite rambunctious. He wanted to touch everything he could see: my adjusting table, my model skeleton, and my glass knick knacks. He couldn't just lie on my table, he had to move constantly. He was up on my table one second and slithered to the floor the next. It was quite an exhausting session for all involved, but we were able to muscle test him and identify substances that made his otherwise strong muscles weak. I sent him and his family home with instructions of what to put into his environment and diet and what to remove. Two weeks later, he returned a different kid. He was still chatty, but now he was focused and calm. His mom reported that out of all the substances we tested, within minutes of ingesting food dyes he consistently lost focus and control. I've noticed this in adults as well.

If you have ever seen a fruit tray you can appreciate the beautiful colors that Mother Nature offers for a healthy diet. Food dyes, on the other hand, are all kinds of trouble. Reported in the October 2010 *Journal of Environmental Health Perspectives*, food dyes have a connection to behavioral problems, hypersensitivity reactions and cancer. Foods with food dyes should be avoided. This is another reason to read nutritional labels.

If the label has "artificial colors" listed, you know to avoid it. Other terms to avoid include the actual color that is added like blue, green, red or yellow — often with a number after it like "yellow 6." Other terms like, FD&C Lakes, are also indications that artificial colors have been added.

Safer colors in foods come from beets, oranges, lycopene from tomatoes, spinach, and turmeric. These are acceptable colors to see on a food label.

ARTIFICIAL FLAVORS

We like food to taste good, and the companies that create processed food bring in specialized scientists to combine just the right amount of chemicals from petroleum and other nonedible substances to entice us to eat their product and purchase it again and again. These artificial flavors are created in a laboratory and can contribute to adverse effects in some people, like dizziness, headaches, and fatigue.

Natural flavors are not much better. Also created in a laboratory, natural flavors come from natural substances like spices, fruit, vegetables, plants, or any food (even fish, chicken or beef) in addition to chemicals. Try to avoid both but certainly the artificial flavors. If you are allergic to MSG—a flavor enhancer—avoid foods with labels that list monosodium glutamate.

"NATURAL"

When you see the word "natural" on a product, what do you think it means? Most people think it means an absence of synthetic chemicals, artificial ingredients, and preservatives. Some people think it means organic. It actually doesn't necessarily mean any of these things since the FDA chose not to make any official definition of the term "natural." It can mean whatever the manufacturer wants the population to perceive their product as.

Most "natural" flavors contain dangerous chemical solvents and preservatives so it's best to avoid them.

PRESERVATIVES

Anything in a box or a bag that needs to have "shelf life" will have preservatives. They keep products tasting fresh, prevent the growth of bacteria, and, in many cases, prevent mold. Unfortunately they also can have negative effects on health. Here are the ones to watch out for:

- Sodium nitrite
- Carrageenan
- Sodium benzoate

This is why The Supercharged Method includes cleaning the cupboards and restocking the kitchen. If this seems too daunting or you feel you aren't ready, I've included some temporary substitutes or better alternatives. Some safer store-bought items are often labeled paleo friendly or Whole 30 friendly. Recipes that are labeled paleo, Whole 30, or keto friendly will not have artificial flavors, colors, dangerous oils, or sugar and are typically safe to eat. I have stevia and monk fruit as alternatives to sugar but sugar alcohols are acceptable as well, as long as they agree with your digestive tract and don't cause gas or bloating. Try to buy organic when possible and refer to the website www.EWG.org for the latest dirty dozen and clean fifteen list of produce with the most (dirty) and the least (clean) pesticides. And most of all remember this: Chips, cookies, and crackers are designed to make you overeat. Next meal, go back to your whole foods. No blame or shame. Let the junk be an exception and the good stuff be your default.

DETOX FROM CAFFEINE AND ALCOHOL

I know you heard me hint about this topic in the introduction. If you thought I forgot about it, I didn't. It's time to bite the bullet and step away from the two vices that most of my patients have a hard time giving up. Their coffee and their wine. You can try to convince me all day long that you can't live without it and that it has been shown to have antioxidants and so much more but I will tell you that once you are off caffeine and alcohol you will understand why I am so adamant about removing them from your diet.

Caffeine and alcohol often affect not only your energy, clarity, and focus but also your sleep, your mood, your brain, and your gut. Caffeine is often used to increase energy, focus, and clarity, but in some people, or if over used, it can cause negative effects.

It will take a good two weeks to get over the withdrawal. Drink more water than usual, take a half teaspoon of sea salt if you get a headache and be patient. The sea salt will provide electrolytes that often can help you get over that hump. You can wean yourself off over a longer period of time or just pick a date and stop. It's hard, I know. But you can do hard things. I'm sure some of you have taken hard classes, gotten degrees, gone into the military, delivered babies, held down multiple jobs—you know how to do hard things and you can do this. After going off caffeine for our 10-Day Supercharged Cleanse, Jill, my office manager felt so good she chose not to go back to her daily caffeine fix. This is the hardest part of the program. If you can do this the rest is a breeze.

CAFFEINE	ALCOHOL
After an initial burst of energy, it can cause fatigue once it is metabolized.	Alcohol can affect sleep by disrupting REM sleep.
Consider that it may be the added sugar or honey you use to sweeten your coffee that may be causing a blood sugar imbalance causing you to be tired or "foggy brained."	It decreases the neurotransmitter serotonin which can result in poor sleep and poor mood.
Coffee is known for its mold contamination, which many people are sensitive to.	Alcohol inhibits the absorption of B12, folate, and zinc, all vital for energy, clarity, and focus.
Caffeine increases the levels of the hormones epinephrine and cortisol, contributing to a "stressed out" feeling.	Alcohol can contribute to dehydration and rob you of vitamins and minerals needed for energy production and other metabolic functions.
Withdrawal from caffeine can cause fatigue, irritability, and inability to concentrate.	It increases uric acid which can contribute to gout in some people.
Caffeine can interfere with sleep quality.	It can cause blood sugar imbalances.
Caffeine can contribute to ulcers and gastritis.	Alcohol causes an inflammatory reaction in the gastrointestinal system.

Go off alcohol and caffeine while you are doing The Super-charged Method. Give yourself up to two weeks to detox, reducing your intake slowly to avoid withdrawal symptoms. You may be surprised how much better you feel once you have been off them for a while.

CHAPTER HIGHLIGHTS

★ Avoid processed foods.

★ Avoid high fructose corn syrup and other sugars.

★ Avoid artificial sweeteners, colors, and flavors.

★ Avoid preservatives.

★ Fructose damages the lining of the blood vessels and intestines.

★ Choose healthy whole foods and sweeteners.

★ Use www.EWG.org as a resource.

★ Caffeine and alcohol often affect not only your energy, clarity, and focus but also your sleep, your mood, your brain, and your gut.

SECTION TWO

DRINK UP

"Hey you. Drink some water."

—Dr. Stacey

CHAPTER 3

HYDRATION

THE IMPORTANCE OF HYDRATION

The body cannot function properly without water. Water helps transport vitamins, minerals, neurotransmitters, hormones, essential nutrients, and oxygen throughout the body. It helps maintain a healthy heart rate and blood pressure and regulates body temperature. Water helps with detoxification and waste removal through the liver, kidneys, intestinal tract, and skin. It also helps create saliva in the mouth which helps you digest carbohydrates, balance the bacteria that naturally resides there, and keeps your teeth healthy.

I have a patient that had his saliva glands removed on one side of his mouth. He has to work hard to keep his mouth hydrated because a dry mouth has impaired his ability to keep his teeth healthy on that side.

A well hydrated body can flush out toxins and waste products that would otherwise damage the tissues of the body. The kidneys work to filter toxins exposed to the body, and removing them from the body is important for optimal health. The bowel also needs water to remove toxins from your digestive system and allow for healthy movement through the intestines.

Water also allows for better regulation of body temperature. Sweating when you are too hot allows the body to cool down. When the body gets overheated you might experience dizziness, confusion, and nausea. If this goes untreated, the body can go into shock which could be fatal.

Did you know that the discs of your spine are like little cushions that act like shock absorbers? These discs need water to maintain their structure and work properly. Many people notice that their back pain improves when they are well hydrated. This goes for joints like your knees as well.

Adequate hydration is important for cognitive function. Being dehydrated by just 2% can cause a decrease in attention and memory. That means you won't even be thirsty when your mind starts wandering. Drinking water throughout the day can help your brain function at its best. Hydration is especially important for high level athletes because it can affect strength, power and endurance.

Another important reason to drink water is it helps you balance your blood pressure. Dehydration can restrict blood flow causing your blood pressure to drop and make you feel cold. This can cause a decrease in blood flow to your brain. Without adequate blood flow to the brain you will feel exhausted. If your blood pressure drops too low, you may get dizzy, black out, and fall down. Low blood pressure is typically lower than 90/60 mm/ Hg, if you know where yours typically stands, or, if you have the symptoms just described, you may want to have it checked. Your brain is made of fat and water. In fact, 73% of your brain is made of water. When you are dehydrated your brain can temporarily shrink. This can contribute to headaches in some people.

A 2003 study in the *Journal of Clinical Endocrinology and Metabolism* showed that drinking just over 16 ounces of water increased a person's metabolic rate within ten to 40 minutes by approximately 30%. Since a higher metabolic rate can burn calories more efficiently, this shows that drinking water can help improve energy and weight loss.

Functions of Hydration:

- Body temperature regulation
- Joint lubrication
- Infection prevention
- Nutrient delivery
- Brain function
- Blood pressure balance
- Detoxification
- Waste removal
- Saliva production

DEHYDRATION

Symptoms of dehydration can occur without feeling thirsty. If you are tired or weak you can be dehydrated. Headaches, dry skin, and constipation are also signs of dehydration. If you look at your tongue in the mirror and see the edges have teeth marks, it can be due to dehydration causing a swollen tongue.

Dehydration can cause decreased sweat production which can impair your ability to remove toxins through your skin and modulate body temperature. It can cause low blood pressure which can put you at risk of getting light headed and fainting. It can also cause a lack of electrolytes that can lead to muscle cramping like those "Charley horses" you get in your legs or feet that wake you up at night.

People at risk of dehydration include athletes or those who sweat a lot when they work out, those with Crohn's disease or colitis, those with undiagnosed celiac disease and non-celiac gluten sensitivity, and people who don't drink enough water (am I looking at you?).

If you are already a water drinker, you know how good you feel when you are well hydrated. Once you start drinking water, you tend to crave it, knowing juice, soda, and coffee just won't cut it. There are a few reasons for this, and if you listen to your body you will find this to be true for you as well.

I once asked a patient how much water she was drinking throughout the week. She told me that if margaritas counted, then I had nothing to worry about. Now, I am partial to a good margarita, but they don't count as part of your water intake. In fact, alcohol is one of the toxins that we want to remove. We get toxins from the food we eat (such as additives and artificial colors and flavors), fluids we drink, medications, cosmetics, shampoos, conditioners, lotions, and detergents. Even the cookware we use and the bottles that hold our drinks leach toxins. Basically, all the things we eat, drink, touch, and breathe.

When these toxins get into our bloodstream they eventually pass through the kidneys which, among other amazing things, filter the blood and send the toxins and waste products in one direction and the minerals, nutrients, hormones, and neurotransmitters in the other. Every ten to 15 seconds a small amount of toxins and waste products get sent from the kidneys down two long tubes to be stored in the bladder. When your bladder feels full and you are near a bathroom, you release them. If you haven't been drinking enough fluids you will notice that your urine is a dark yellow. This is because it is concentrated. The yellow color comes from a pigment called urochrome. When you drink water urochrome gets diluted causing the color of your urine to be paler. Looking at the color of your urine is an excellent way to make sure you are getting enough water. Note that we are not aiming for clear urine, we want a pale yellow instead. If your urine is clear, lower your intake of water.

Side note: When I prescribe B vitamins to a patient I will tell them to watch out for three things. One, if you take them on an empty stomach it can make you nauseous; two, if you take them too close to bedtime it may keep you up because they can give you energy; three, they will turn your urine bright yellow-orange, so don't freak out. This is because there are yellow-orange pigments in some B vitamins. It is not harmful, just shocking to see for the first time.

CHAPTER HIGHLIGHTS

- ★ Water helps transport vitamins, minerals, neurotransmitters, hormones, essential nutrients, and oxygen through the body.
- ★ Drinking water helps maintain a healthy heart rate and blood pressure and regulates body temperature.
- ★ Water helps with detoxification and waste removal through the liver, kidneys, intestinal tract and skin.

★ Being dehydrated by just 2% can cause a decrease in attention and memory.

★ 73% of your brain is made of water. When you are dehydrated your brain can temporarily shrink.

★ Drinking water increases metabolic rate.

★ Looking at the color of your urine is an excellent way to make sure you are getting enough water.

CHAPTER 4

WASTE REMOVAL

The body is brilliant at removing waste. It uses the kidneys, liver, large intestine, lungs, and skin to remove all sorts of waste that would otherwise harm the body.

THE URINARY SYSTEM

The urinary system consists of:

- Kidneys, which actually look like two kidney beans and are located in the middle of your back and filter your blood.
- Ureters, which are two long tubes that move waste products from the kidneys into the bladder.
- Bladder, which is the pouch that holds urine until you are ready to release it.
- Urethra, the tube that allows you to eliminate the toxins and waste products from your body.

Staying well hydrated by drinking water throughout the day will help maintain function of the urinary system.

THE INTESTINAL SYSTEM

Your intestines are another water-dependent, toxin-removing system of the body. Your digestive system is the tube that starts in your mouth, extends to your throat and down your esophagus, continues through your stomach to a long track called your small intestines, and then to your large intestines and out through your rectum.

When you are not drinking enough water, you will not have enough fluid to move the waste products in your large intestines or bowel. Constipation from dehydration will cause the toxins that have been released into the stool to reabsorb through the lining of the intestines if they are sitting in there too long.

I once had a young patient who was around five years old. She was sluggish and had a green tinge to her skin. Her belly was bloated and she was not pooping. Her diet consisted of processed cereal with the lovely hues of artificial coloring that children are so drawn to, processed low quality meats like hot dogs and bologna, and Faygo red pop (soda for you people who don't call it "pop"). I educated her and her parents that some food is nice to look at but not so good for your insides. They changed her diet and switched her from pop to water. Within two weeks she was pooping regularly, bouncing off the walls, happy as a clam, and no longer looked like Mr. Grinch.

Adequate water and fiber work together to keep a healthy digestive system. The fiber from vegetables, fruit, and whole grains expands when you drink water. This complex works like a broom to brush out the intestines of toxins and waste material.

THE SKIN

Sweating is another way we remove toxins. If you sweat heavily, work out to the point of sweating, use a sauna, have hot flashes, or have a medical condition like hyperthyroidism, then you are sweating out toxins, minerals, and water. Some people, like those with a low functioning thyroid, have a hard time sweating. Sweating is an excellent way the body modulates body temperature and releases toxins, but it is equally important to replenish the water lost in the process. If you sweat a lot and your muscles are cramping, try adding a half a teaspoon of sea salt or an electrolyte blend to your water since the loss of water can take with it many minerals you need to contract and relax your muscles.

CHAPTER HIGHLIGHTS

★ The kidneys, liver, large intestine, lungs, and skin remove waste products from the body.

★ Drinking water throughout the day will help maintain function of the urinary system.

★ Drink water to move the waste products through your large intestines or bowel.

★ Adequate water and fiber work together to keep a healthy digestive system.

★ Sweating is an excellent way the body modulates body temperature and releases toxins, but it is equally important to replenish the water lost in the process.

★ If you sweat a lot and your muscles are cramping, try adding a half a teaspoon of sea salt or an electrolyte blend to your water.

CHAPTER 5

GETTING IT DOWN

Are you someone who easily drinks water all day or are you someone who can go days without even a sip? It may seem like you can get what you need from the food you eat and various drinks but sooner or later it will catch up to you. If you are struggling with your health and are not drinking water, consider starting now.

HOW MUCH WATER TO DRINK

There are great debates on how much water you should drink in a day. All bodies are different, but we all function best when we drink water. If you are drinking nothing all day and just consuming food, start with six cups of water a day and move up from there. If you are drinking caffeinated and sugary drinks, start by replacing some of them, then all of them. (Okay gremlins, you can keep your one cup of coffee a day, sheesh, but consume it before noon.) If you want to get the most out of a hydrated body, drink half of your body weight in ounces of water a day. That means if you weigh 160 pounds, drink 80 ounces of water a day. Although coffee, caffeinated tea, sugared or artificially sweetened soda, and juice do not count toward your water intake; water with electrolytes or flavored naturally does.

HOW TO DRINK MORE WATER

If you are not a water drinker there are many tips and tricks you can use to get your quota of water for the day.

A patient who had embarked on The Supercharged Method was a self-proclaimed "water hater." She told me that water just didn't agree with her. I gave her some suggestions, and when she returned she shared her water routine with me. I liked it so much I adopted it for myself. Here is that routine and an explanation as to why I like the different components of it.

Within 30 minutes of waking, fill a 32-ounce (quart-sized) Mason jar with two stevia/erythritol packets, the juice of half a lime or lemon, and fill with cold water. Stick in a silicone straw. Consume within an hour. Do this again in the evening.

You can alternatively use dehydrated lemon or lime and other natural zero-calorie sweeteners like monk fruit. Evaluate how your belly likes it. If it causes gas or bloating, switch to another sweetener.

Start Drinking Water within 30 Minutes of Waking

Believe it or not, this is an example of the small wins you will collect to create habits to be successful with The Supercharged Method. It's easy, good for your skin and overall health, makes you more alert and helps you feel accomplished. If you did nothing else all day, at least you drank your morning water. Yay you!

Mason Jars Are Awesome

A Mason jar makes it super easy to know how much you are drinking, they are inexpensive, and I bet you already have one collecting dust in your basement. It has a top that seals tight and doesn't spill when you place it on the passenger seat of your car. The jar is made of glass, not plastic, so we don't have to worry about BPA or phthalates getting into your water from the acidity of the lemon or lime. In fact, plastic water bottles can leach BPA even without any acids present. An alternative would be a stainless steel thermos or tumbler.

The Benefits of Lemons and Limes

Lemon and lime juice in your morning water will make you feel like you are having something of substance so you don't feel as hungry. The diluted juice is also very low on the glycemic index, meaning it will not spike your insulin level. It provides some vitamin C which is a strong antioxidant and a vitamin your body cannot produce itself. Lemons and limes are on the acidic side of the pH scale of zero to 14, being a two, with pure water being a neutral seven. This can be deceiving since the more acidic the body is, the unhealthier it tends to be, and the more alkaline a body is, the healthier it tends to be. Although lemons and limes are acidic, they actually make the body more alkaline. It is confusing, I know. This is because once it becomes metabolized, lemon and lime juice become alkaline with a pH above seven. Potential benefits are lower cholesterol and inflammation, and increased metabolism, immunity, and energy.

Avoid Lemon or Lime Juice If…

- Your teeth become sensitive to hot or cold, or become discolored.
- You have mouth sores, like a canker sore or mouth ulcer.
- You feel any discomfort after drinking.
- You take a medication that may interact with lemon or lime.

Silicone and Glass Straws

Drinking from a straw makes getting the water down so much easier. Don't believe me? Try it. If the straw has a wider diameter, it's even easier. Drinking from a straw will help keep the acidic lemon or lime juice off your teeth, protecting your enamel. I once went to the dentist for a dental cleaning, and after she finished, she looked at me accusingly and said, "Are you chewing on lemons?" I admitted that I was drinking more water with lemon and lime juice in it. Do you know what she told me? Yep, you got it. She said, "Use a straw." If your teeth become discolored or sensitive to hot or cold, discontinue the lemon or lime juice. The straw doesn't have to be silicone. It can be glass or stainless steel as well. Avoid a plastic drinking straw because the acidity of the lemon/lime juice will pull plastic from the straw, and it will enter your drinking water. Glass straws are gorgeous and I love the company, Strawsome. I had the opportunity to meet the owners and tour their shop when they were just starting out. Not only are they sustainable but they are beautiful to boot. Although their glass straws are strong, don't drop them on a hard floor. Silicone straws are also sustainable. They are bendy and can be stored in the smallest of cases for transport.

You can also choose to use a stainless steel straw or forgo a straw altogether.

Natural Sweeteners If You Must

Drink plain filtered water. If you need some help and choose to sweeten your drink use a natural sweetener. Stevia, allulose, monk fruit and erythritol do not raise your blood sugar, they rarely cause any gastrointestinal distress, and make you feel like you are ingesting something substantial enough to keep hunger at bay until it is time to eat. Do not use sucralose/Splenda, aspartame/Equal, saccharin/Sweet-n-Low, agave, sugar, or other fruit juice. Of course it is better to not need to sweeten water to get it down but use it if you need to.

OTHER WATER TIPS AND TRICKS

Use an app. There are great apps that remind you to drink your water—from a cute cartoon plant that you have to water to keep healthy to programmed reminders. Type "drink water" in the search bar of your smart phone's app store and you will see a variety of apps you can use to help you drink more water.

Infuse it. Infusing your water with fruits, vegetables, and herbs can help make the water drinking experience downright enjoyable. To infuse water you can find small baskets or bags to hang in your water that you can fill with a variety of things to flavor it with.

Lemon	Cucumber	Watermelon
Lime	Berries	Orange

Celery	Cilantro	Cayenne
Mint	Cinnamon	Herbal tea
Parsley	Ginger	Apple cider vinegar

Another interesting way to get your daily water in is to make something called Jeera Water. Jeera Water is water infused with cumin and has been used for thousands of years, originating in the Middle East but popular in India. It has a multitude of benefits. Cumin is an herb from the parsley family. You will most commonly find it as seeds or ground spice. A strong anti-inflammatory, it can help reduce pain and discomfort. Rich in antioxidants, it can provide nutrients the body needs to stay healthy. Also known as an antibacterial, cumin or Jeera Water, can help digestion and immunity.

To make Jeera Water you boil two cups of water and then add two heaping teaspoons of cumin seeds. Boil until the liquid is reduced by half. Drain the liquid to drink. You can drink it hot or cold. You can also add cinnamon, citrus zest, or ginger if you'd like.

THE SAFEST WATER TO DRINK

I'm not going to be too particular about the quality of your water if you have been drinking cola for the last 20 years and are now drinking water. But to up your water game, consider investing in a good filter system. If you have city water, it is filtered to a certain extent but can still contain some bacteria, chemicals, heavy metals, and even some medication. Filtered water even tastes better. Bottled water is easy and convenient, but it can be expensive over time and I'm a stickler about avoiding water from plastic containers. BPA from plastics easily gets into the water with temperature changes and can cause all sorts of hormonal problems and, potentially, cancer. Purchasing water in glass containers is acceptable but expensive. I recommend a home filtration unit that can clean the water you drink, the water you cook with, and the water you bathe with as well.

WORKSHEET ONE: TAKING INVENTORY

To use this chart you can either fill in the star when you have completed a day of eight glasses of water or you can shade in a point in the star for every glass of water you drink throughout the day.

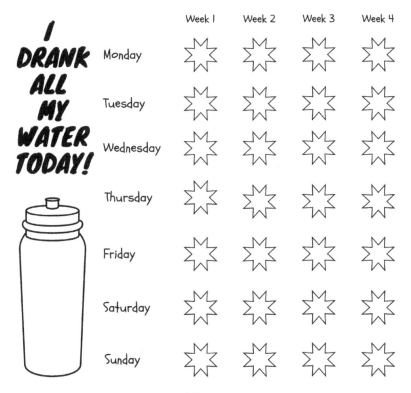

Two Special Recipes (for when you are craving a cocktail or a soda)

Lemon Ginger Mocktail:

- 2 ounces ginger juice homemade or store bought
- 2 ounces lemon juice fresh pressed
- Soda water to taste
- Ice
- Fresh ginger
- Optional: Stevia or monk fruit to taste
- Optional: rub the rim of the glass with the fresh piece of ginger.

Pour lemon juice and ginger juice in a cocktail shaker and add an ice cube. Close the lid tightly and shake for about 15 seconds. Add natural zero-sugar sweetener to taste. Pour into martini glass. Top with soda water and decorate with a piece of fresh ginger.

Zero Sugar Fruity Soda

- 12 fluid ounces of sparkling water
- One serving of Ultima Replenisher or other zero-sugar, naturally sweetened drink mix or electolyte blend.

Fill a tall glass with ice cubes. Pour drink mix and sparkling water into glass. Enjoy. Ultima Replenisher comes in flavors of cherry, raspberry, lemon, orange, grape and more.

Benjamin, my older son, remembers taking lunch to school in glass containers and watching other kids eat sandwiches with bread "as white as snow" while he brought leftovers. He remembers growing up without a microwave. Being a parent is not easy. There is no guidebook. We practice on our kids and figure it out as we go. He may have felt captive to my "natural food" ways but when he remembers that he learned to cook at a young age and now cooks sought-after dishes for his community, I hear pride in his voice. When I asked him what he is spending his money on these days, one of the items he lists is organic vegetables. I smile. Go ahead, be that parent that wants the best for your kids' health. They might balk but they are paying attention.

CHAPTER HIGHLIGHTS

★ Drink half of your body weight in ounces of water a day.

★ Consume a good amount of your daily water in the morning.

★ Drink out of glass or stainless steel containers. Avoid plastics.

★ Flavor water with fruit, vegetables, herbs, herbal teas, and spices.

★ Try using a silicone, stainless steel, or glass straw.

★ Invest in a good water filtration system.

★ Action Task: Make four quart Mason jars of water and keep in the refrigerator to consume over the day.

SECTION THREE

SLEEP BETTER

"Some people can't sleep because they have insomnia.
I can't sleep because I have internet."

—Anonymous

CHAPTER 6

BEAUTY SLEEP

Where we once thought sleep was this void of mental activity we now know that isn't the case. Our brain actually gets a workout when we sleep. Brain cells communicate with each other and with nerve cells throughout the spinal cord through chemical compounds called neurotransmitters. These chemicals signal when to be awake and alert, and when not to.

There are five stages of sleep. Stage one is a light sleep where our eyes are moving slowly, and our muscle activity slows down. Stage two is where our eye movements stop, and the electrical activity in our brain slows down. In stage three, the brain alternates between fast and slow waves. The slow waves are called delta waves. Stage four is exclusively delta waves and is considered "deep sleep." There is no eye movement or muscle activity during deep sleep. The last stage is REM sleep. Rapid eye movements, a change in breathing and the arms and legs becoming temporarily paralyzed are characteristics of REM sleep. Being paralyzed even temporarily sounds scary, but it is important to keep us from getting up unknowingly and potentially hurting ourselves. This is often where bizarre dreams occur.

Since food and chemicals affect neurotransmitter function, food and chemicals affect sleep as well. Compounds that can cause sleep issues include caffeine, decongestants, antidepressants, sugar, nicotine and alcohol.

It's important to get enough sleep. Adults need anywhere from six to nine hours of sleep a night. One night of poor sleep can throw your sleep patterns off for the next night or two, so it's important to stay consistent with bedtime routines.

Studies have shown that sleep deprivation is dangerous and a common cause of car accidents. You can't focus or think clearly when you are sleep deprived. Some people notice the effects of sleep deprivation more quickly than others. If you are drowsy, have trouble keeping your eyes open, can't concentrate, or feel like your brain is full of cotton or foggy, you most likely need more sleep.

Biological Impact of Sleep

The nervous system repairs itself during sleep. Many byproducts of normal cellular activity are created when we are awake. Sleep allows us to clean up these byproducts before they cause damage. Sleep also activates areas of brain function that haven't been adequately used during the day, keeping these areas healthy.

Increased cellular production of protein happens when you sleep. This is important for tissue repair, growth of muscle, and healing.

Areas in the brain detect light and tell us when to wake and when to sleep. When light starts fading our bodies release a hormone called melatonin which makes us feel drowsy and ready to sleep. Production of melatonin stops when light hits the back of our eyes and sends messages to our brain signaling that it is time to wake up.

People who work nights or are on shift work are at risk for sleep issues and other symptoms associated with sleep disturbance such as digestive issues, increased risk of cardiovascular problems, and emotional and mental issues.

CREATING HEALTHY SLEEP HABITS

Being consistent with when you go to sleep and when you wake up is important to healthy sleep. You can actually train your body to fall asleep at a certain time and wake up at a certain time if you are consistent and mindful of factors that will interfere with good sleep. If you do nothing else regarding your sleep, at least make a point to go to sleep and wake up at the same time consistently.

Staying away from screens (phones, laptops, television) an hour to a few hours before bed will help your brain get ready for rest. We often fill our brains with stimulation right before bed and expect to get to sleep. Then we are up counting sheep.

Avoid eating or drinking two to three hours before bed, including alcohol.

Exercise daily.

Work with your circadian rhythm by getting outside in the morning when it's light and winding down when the sun goes down.

Expose yourself to full-spectrum bright light in the early morning.

Consider meditation, guided imagery or journaling. When your mind's going a mile a minute thinking of all the things you have to do or don't want to forget, journaling can help empty your mind. If you're someone with a long to-do list, write it down in your journal. This can give you comfort knowing you can reflect on your tasks in the morning since they are down on paper. Even stressful thoughts dissipate easier when they are written down. You can even write down what you would like to see happen to those stressful situations if you had a magic wand. Your brain will rest easier when you have something productive planned even if it's not realistically possible. Your brain will be more at ease.

An exercise in relieving stress:

Take out a piece of paper and a pen. Write down all the issues causing you stress. Under each of them list every emotion you can think of that that issue evokes. You may have to really imagine yourself back in the situation to distinguish what it is that you feel. Write it all down. When that is complete, rest for 15 minutes. Just let your mind go blank. It won't be that hard since you just used a lot of brain power pulling out all those feelings. When you have rested for 15 minutes reflect once more on the issues and add any other feelings that you missed the first time around. Once you have listed every feeling that each issue brings up in you, rest again for 15 minutes. Now go about your day or go to sleep and notice if you feel less stressed about those issues or if productive solutions appear when they didn't before when so much emotion was attached.

Consider herbs and supplements for better sleep. (Do not take herbs or supplements with any medications without talking to your doctor first.)

Nutritional sleep aids:

- 5 Hydroxytryptophan (Do not take with SSRIs)
- Ashwagandha (200 mg twice a day)
- B Complex (taken early in the day)
- L-Theanine
- L-Tryptophan
- Magnesium citrate or glycinate
- GABA
- Tulsi (Holy Basil)
- Melatonin (sustained release or topical)
- Phosphatidylserine
- CBD/Hemp oil
- Valerian Root
- Wild Yam (topically)

Other sleep aids:

- Blue light blockers
- Darkness
- Epsom salt baths
- Lavender essential oil

Write up a plan and commitment to sleep. Commit to a time for turning off electronics and to gently stretch, practice yoga, read, meditate, or listen to soft music. Write down all the bad thoughts, worries, things to do, and concerns you have that would keep you from sleeping. This is called a "brain dump." When that is completed, turn off the lights and close your eyes.

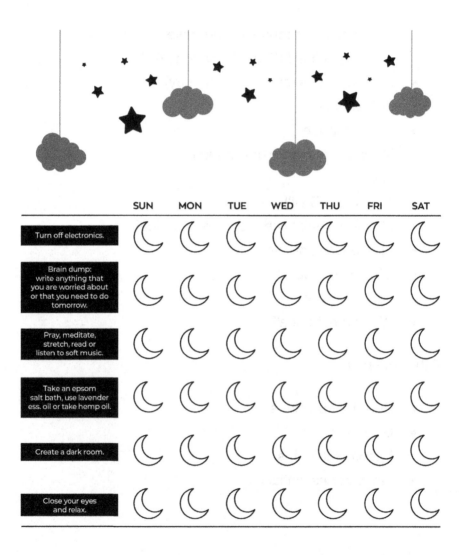

	SUN	MON	TUE	WED	THU	FRI	SAT
Turn off electronics.	☾	☾	☾	☾	☾	☾	☾
Brain dump: write anything that you are worried about or that you need to do tomorrow.	☾	☾	☾	☾	☾	☾	☾
Pray, meditate, stretch, read or listen to soft music.	☾	☾	☾	☾	☾	☾	☾
Take an epsom salt bath, use lavender ess. oil or take hemp oil.	☾	☾	☾	☾	☾	☾	☾
Create a dark room.	☾	☾	☾	☾	☾	☾	☾
Close your eyes and relax.	☾	☾	☾	☾	☾	☾	☾

Good sleep is important, and it may take some time to find your magical combination of things to do and things to avoid. It may be a decrease in sugar, caffeine, and alcohol, or eliminating them altogether. It may be a combination of ashwagandha and CBD oil. It may even be finding a practitioner to help balance your hormones. Whatever it is, don't stop investigating until you have consistent good restorative sleep. It's that important.

CHAPTER HIGHLIGHTS

- ★ There are five stages of sleep.
- ★ Food and chemicals affect sleep.
- ★ Adults need anywhere from six to nine hours of sleep a night.
- ★ Sleep deprivation is dangerous and a common cause of car accidents.
- ★ The nervous system repairs itself during sleep.
- ★ Melatonin is a hormone that makes us feel drowsy and ready to sleep.
- ★ Be consistent with when you go to sleep and when you wake.
- ★ Avoid eating, drinking, and screen time three hours before bed.
- ★ Expose yourself to full-spectrum bright light in the early morning.
- ★ There are many natural sleep aids. If needed, choose the ones that work for you.

CHAPTER 7

CAUSES FOR INSOMNIA

Whether you have trouble falling asleep or staying asleep, insomnia needs to be resolved. Often sleep medication will not allow you to get the restorative sleep that is necessary to avoid the side effects of sleep deprivation. Get to the root cause and develop good sleep hygiene so medication won't be necessary. Don't be discouraged if it takes some time and different combinations to figure out your magic formula for sleep.

The following can all cause poor sleep:

- Artificial light
- Electronic devices and overstimulation
- Fast-paced lifestyle
- Chronic underlying stress/worry/ deadlines

STRESS

Stress is a major contributor to sleep problems. Please don't step over this issue. Stress can be at the root of many health conditions and needs to be addressed. It may be emotional, where you would benefit from seeing a therapist, journaling, meditating, walking, identifying and correcting for adrenal imbalances, exercising or delegating authority when you are burning the candle at both ends. Whatever is contributing to your stress needs to be resolved, even if it's just the way you think about the situation. If your brain thinks something is an opportunity or a lesson instead of a stressful burden, it may give you a chance to rest and catch up.

Stress can show itself as a chronic sleep problem. Stress is good when it challenges our bodies and souls, but too much can cause a host of problems including sleep issues. It's always a good idea to check in with your doctor and share the stress you are under. Together you can decide if you are juggling your stress well or if you need added support.

Illnesses that can cause sleep issues:

- Depression
- Anxiety
- Bipolar disorder
- Post Traumatic Stress Disorder (PTSD)
- Substance abuse
- Heart disease
- Chronic pain
- Diabetes
- Hormonal imbalances
- Hyperthyroidism

DISRUPTIONS

Disruptions of your circadian rhythm will also interrupt restorative sleep. If you are traveling across time zones, working the night shift, frequently changing work shifts or exposed to blue light from your computer or phone, find a way to regulate your sleep cycle and do that consistently.

BLUE LIGHT

Let's talk about blue light for a moment. Raise your hand if your downtime before bed includes you scrolling through your phone. Yep. It's pretty common. Blue light, combined with all the other colors of the rainbow, comes from the white light that the sun gives off. That is our main source of blue light. Fluorescent bulbs, often found in overhead ceiling lights in basements and offices, and LED lights in your smartphone, tablet and TV screen also emit blue light. A 2011 study published in the *Journal of Applied Physiology* showed that all light suppresses melatonin in humans (this is why you want a dark room to sleep in) with the short-wavelength that is blue light causing the most suppression of melatonin (which disrupts circadian rhythm and can result in a decrease in alertness and performance). Limit your blue light exposure to the daylight and up until one to three hours before bed. If you can't do that, there are glasses with lenses tinted amber that may be able to block the blue light and subsequently block the melatonin drop. The jury is still out on their effectiveness, but they are safe enough to experiment with and compare your sleep when using them to sleep after avoiding blue light for one to three hours before bed. Go without blue light for at least an hour before bed for a few weeks and evaluate your sleep.

STIMULANTS AND DEPRESSANTS

Caffeine intake is a very common cause of insomnia. Not only is caffeine found in expected sources like coffee and tea, caffeine can also be found in significant amounts in chocolate, energy drinks, some supplements, and some medication. Remove all stimulants from your diet for two weeks. This is an important action step to take if you are having trouble sleeping. Even that one sip of coffee in the morning or that chocolate chip cookie in the evening can contribute to poor sleep. In a 2017 review of multiple studies in the journal *Sleep Medicine Reviews*, caffeine typically prolonged the time it took to go from fully awake to asleep, reduced total sleep time and impaired sleep quality.

Alcohol can impair sleep. The central nervous system consists of your brain and spinal cord. Messages are constantly being relayed through this system such as thoughts, movements, awareness of surroundings, temperature changes and threats, among others. Alcohol is a central nervous system depressant. It slows down the messages of all this important communication. This slowing down is sedating to the brain. That is why many people use alcohol before bed to get to sleep. However, alcohol use before bed can cause poor sleep quality and sleep disturbances.

Sugar is used as a pick-me-up when your body is tired but you choose to stay up instead of going to sleep. Sugar is a stimulant that activates neurotransmitters in the brain. These neurotransmitters release chemicals that make you feel happy and awake. Sugar was shown to disrupt sleep in a 2016 study demonstrating that people with a diet high in sugar were associated with lighter, less restorative sleep and more frequent waking. When you eat sugar your blood sugar will spike. This spike can be a stimulant and keep you up later than your body would normally signal you to go to sleep. Sugar can cause a spike and crash of blood sugar that can make you hungry in the middle of the night or early morning, causing you to wake up before you have had enough rest. Additionally, sugar needs magnesium to be processed by your body, which can cause a deficiency in this mineral—a mineral that helps you relax.

Eating too late at night can cause reflux in people who are prone to it. In my own clinic, patients have noticed that they sleep better and wake up less hungry when they stop eating three hours before bed but not longer.

Medications can cause insomnia. Are you taking medication that is causing you to lose sleep? If you are, talk to your prescribing doctor. If the medication is affecting your sleep there may be an alternative. Never go off medication without talking to your doctor. Examples of the medications that impact sleep are in the parentheses, but there are other medications that can be in that category.

- Alpha-blockers (Cardura, Flomax)
- Beta-blockers (Coreg, Lopressor, Toprol)
- Corticosteroids (Cortisol, Prednisone, Medrol)

- SSRI antidepressants (Celexa, Prozac, Lexapro, Serafem, Paxil, Luvox, Zoloft)
- ACE Inhibitors (Lotensin, Vasotec, Lisinopril)
- ARBs (Losartan, Valsartan)
- Cholinesterase inhibitors (Aricept, Razadyne)
- H1 antagonists (Zyrtec, Claritin, Allegra, Xyzal)
- Statins (Lipitor, Mevacor, Crestor, Zocor, Atorvastatin, Simvastatin)

Supplements can sometimes cause insomnia if taken too close to bedtime or even earlier if you are sensitive to their stimulating effects. If this is the case for you, try to take these supplements before noon. Here are a few that can stimulate you:

Adrenal glandulars	Glucosamine/chondroitin
B Vitamins	Green Tea
Caffeine	Guarana
Ginseng	Vitamin D

Vitamins can also contribute to insomnia if you have a deficiency in them. A deficiency in Vitamins C, D, and E can cause insomnia as can a deficiency in B vitamins.

MEDICAL CONDITIONS

Medical conditions can impair sleep. Sleep apnea, hyperthyroidism or over-prescribed hypothyroidism, hormonal fluctuations, chronic pain, and anxiety can all affect sleep.

SLEEP APNEA

If you ever watch someone sleep and they seem to not be breathing but then take a deep gasp for air, they may have sleep apnea. Sleep apnea occurs when oxygen cannot adequately get to the lungs and brain during sleep. Often a result of obesity, the buildup of fat around the throat can cause interrupted breathing, as can a weakening of muscles from aging. This can cause the windpipe to collapse, and snoring may occur, which is one of the signs of sleep apnea. When the airflow is cut off from a collapsed windpipe, the lack of oxygen to the brain will cause the sleeping person to awaken just enough to tighten the muscles needed to get in a gasp of air but not enough to actually wake them up. This can happen hundreds of times a night with disastrous effects.

Symptoms of sleep apnea include:

Brain fog

Fatigue

Snoring

High blood pressure

Poor concentration and focus

Episodes of interrupted breathing during sleep

Waking suddenly with a gasp, snort, or choke

Low sex drive

Depression, anxiety, irritability, anger

Morning dry mouth or sore throat

Headaches, most commonly in the morning

Long term effects of sleep apnea include:

Diabetes	Heart failure
High blood pressure	Memory loss
Stroke	Asthma
Tachycardia	Susceptibility to infection
Atrial fibrillation	Fatty liver disease
Heart attack	High cholesterol

It takes a sleep study of overnight monitoring to diagnose and discover the severity of sleep apnea. At that point your doctor may recommend therapy.

Treatments for sleep apnea may include;

- Weight loss
- Quitting smoking
- Allergy treatments
- An oral device to keep the airway open
- Treatment for cardiac or neuromuscular issues
- An airway pressure device that forces air into your nose and mouth

These pressure devices are called CPAP (Continuous Positive Airway Pressure) or BPAP (Bilevel Positive Airway Pressure) machines.

If you think that you have sleep apnea, consult with your doctor and resolve it as soon as possible to avoid the many consequences of sleep deprivation and oxygen deprivation.

NARCOLEPSY

When Josie came in she told me how tired she was. As I listened I made a mental checklist of the questions I wanted to ask and the tests I wanted her to have. She told me she gets sleepy while driving. Since this sounded familiar to my own past situation, I wondered about thyroid, anemia, and blood sugar imbalance. Then she told me that she almost fell asleep while bike riding. This was surprising. It's not uncommon to get sleepy while driving because so much of driving is automatic, but it takes more awareness to bike and your heart rate increases which typically keeps you alert. Then she told me that she actually fell asleep while running on the treadmill, fell, and hurt herself. I asked if she had ever been diagnosed with narcolepsy, a condition that causes excessive daytime sleepiness. She told me that her last doctor had also mentioned it.

Not all fatigue is typical. Fatigue can come from more uncommon sources such as environmental toxins, latent or active viruses, heavy metal toxicity, parasites or other microbial infections, and so much more—including narcolepsy.

Symptoms of narcolepsy include:

- Falling asleep suddenly, anywhere at anytime
- Loss of clarity and focus
- Muscle weakness
- Moments of inability to move or speak
- Hallucinations

Having these symptoms can be frightening and requires medical care. Although in the United States narcolepsy only affects approximately one in 2,000 people, that number may be under-reported.

It may be due to genetics, a chronic virus, or autoimmunity. All the causes seem to involve decreased levels of a chemical in the brain called hypocretin. Hypocretin helps induce sleep, particularly deep REM sleep, and the ability to stay awake.

Treatment is varied and should be under the care of a doctor, but pay attention to the following lifestyle factors: avoid caffeine and alcohol, take naps, stay hydrated, identify and correct any nutrient deficiencies such as iron or B vitamins, and get a healthy amount of quality sleep.

A 2010 study in the *Nevada Journal of Public Health* identified the connection between a low carbohydrate diet and lowering fatigue. So choosing low glycemic foods is another lifestyle habit to implement with this condition.

BACK PAIN

As a chiropractor, I have seen many cases of back pain disrupt sleep. If you can't get comfortable you will not be able to relax enough to get a good night's sleep. Many patients tell me their pain wakes them out of a deep sleep. Back pain is one of the most common reasons people seek out a chiropractor. Chiropractic is also one of the best ways to resolve back pain in order to get good rest. A chiropractic adjustment, which is a movement of a joint manually or with a specialized instrument, allows the return of proper movement to the joint. It is safe and effective when done by a qualified chiropractor. (I don't want to see your five year old walking on your back.)

Putting a pillow between your knees is another way that you can decrease back pain while you are sleeping. When the legs pull on the hip joints, it can cause a misalignment in the pelvis that a pillow between the knees can sometimes help.

Stretch your hamstrings and your butt muscles, or better yet, roll on a foam roller or tennis ball. When you don't feel pain, start exercising and stretching all your muscles attached to your pelvis. It may be tender when you are stretching your muscles but lengthening them can relieve tension in the back, allowing you to have a restful sleep. When you feel better start exercising. Exercising, stretching, and eating whole foods that support your body are a great combination.

Change your mattress. If your mattress is too hard or too soft it can contribute to back pain. Over time your mattress may change shape and may also contribute to back pain. It's time to change your mattress if it is sagging, you can no longer get comfortable in bed, or you sleep better on a different mattress. The National Sleep Foundation recommends replacing your mattress every six to eight years.

HORMONAL IMBALANCE

If you have an overactive thyroid, the excess T3 hormone can contribute to insomnia. If you are under stress, high cortisol levels can keep you alert and anxious, causing you to lose sleep. If you have low progesterone or low DHEA you may have trouble sleeping. Other hormone imbalances can affect sleep as well.

CONSEQUENCES OF SLEEP DEPRIVATION

Sleep deprivation leads to a bunch of issues that lead to a bunch of other issues. It can cause an imbalance in the hormones that regulate hunger (ghrelin and leptin) resulting in increased hunger. When you are overly hungry you often eat foods that are not good for you. A few hundred chip bags and candy wrappers later, you may be dealing with obesity. A lack of sleep causes increased fatigue which will make you lethargic, unfocused, unproductive, and can lead to depression. Sleep deprivation can also increase stress hormones which can affect mood and concentration.

Develop good sleep habits by going to bed at the same time and waking up at the same time, avoiding activities that can impair your sleep and adopting habits that can help.

Before bed avoid:

- Stress
- Heavy foods
- Sugar
- Alcohol
- Caffeine
- Exercise

Instead of looking at electronic screens or your phone choose relaxing activities such as the following:

- Peaceful and loving conversations
- Stretching or foam rolling

- Deep breathing
- Meditating
- Board games
- Crossword puzzles or sudoku
- Coloring
- Journaling
- Reading poetry
- Reading happy and relaxing material
- Writing down what makes you feel grateful
- Taking an (Epsom salt) bath
- Daily reflection, spiritual practice or praying

Don't allow poor sleep to stress you out. If you have a hard time falling asleep, staying asleep or if you find yourself up at 3 a.m., don't sweat it. Get up and practice any of the actions above to keep yourself in a rested state and take a 20-minute nap in the afternoon if needed.

CHAPTER HIGHLIGHTS

★ Get to the root cause of trouble sleeping and develop good sleep hygiene so medication won't be necessary.

★ Stress is good when it challenges our bodies and souls, but too much can cause a host of problems including sleep issues.

★ All light suppresses melatonin in humans with the short-wavelength that is blue light causing the most suppression.

★ Remove all stimulants from your diet.

★ Alcohol use before bed can cause poor sleep quality and sleep disturbances.

★ Some medications and supplements can cause insomnia.

★ Sleep apnea occurs when oxygen cannot adequately get to the lungs and brain during sleep.

★ Back pain can disrupt sleep. See your chiropractor.

★ Narcolepsy may be due to genetics, a chronic virus, or autoimmunity.

★ An overactive thyroid can cause sleep issues.

★ Sleep deprivation can cause an imbalance in the hormones that regulate hunger (ghrelin and leptin) resulting in increased hunger.

SECTION FOUR

EAT RIGHT FOR YOUR LIFE

"When diet is wrong, medicine is of no use.
When diet is correct, medicine is of no need."

—Ayurvedic Proverb

CHAPTER 8

EATING TO BALANCE BLOOD SUGAR

Whether your blood work shows a blood sugar imbalance or not, the way I'm going to teach you to eat will improve your health and may resolve symptoms that you didn't realize you could resolve.

When Anna did The Supercharged Method she had a result she never expected. She came in feeling tired all the time. She couldn't focus at work and was worried her boss was noticing. She incorporated the following steps to improve her blood sugar balance and found that not only did she regain her energy and focus, but she got pregnant after trying unsuccessfully for over four years.

I know you sometimes feel like Pooh Bear with your head full of fluff. The Supercharged Method will help you unfluff your tired brain, and it starts with balancing blood sugar and getting the right nutrients, in sufficient amounts. A random vegetable here and there isn't going to repair the damage that 20 years of eating daily donuts has caused. Balancing your blood sugar will allow you to reclaim your energy, clarity, and focus. This Supercharged Method will provide you the tools to eat in a way that will help you increase your concentration, memory, and critical thinking skills.

When we talk about balancing blood sugar we're looking to eat food that will give us all the nutrients we need. Plus we want to space it out in a way that allows for our insulin to decrease, our G.I. system to digest, and we want to eat often enough that we're not absolutely starving for our next meal and reaching for something sugary.

The rules are simple...one, two, three, or four in 12:

1+2
Every 3-4
in 12

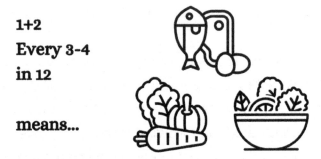

means...

1 serving of protein
plus
2 servings of vegetables
eaten every 3 to 4 hours,
in a 12 hour time frame.

Remember the 1+2 every 3–4 in 12 method? Here we are going to dive deep into the details.

Eat one serving of protein (approximately 15-30 grams or the size of your palm for wild-caught or grass-fed fish, chicken, or beef) and two servings of low glycemic vegetables (above the ground, not including corn; one serving is equal to one half to one cup) every three to four hours in a twelve-hour time frame. From there you can add to these meals: up to two fruits per day (half cup is a serving, one of which should be berries), up to two heavier carbohydrates a day (under the ground vegetables, grains, and corn, half cup per serving) and four servings of healthy fats or oils a day (one serving is one tablespoon).

Now let's take that information and go into some detail.

ONE SERVING OF PROTEIN AT EVERY MEAL.

Choose one serving of protein per meal. Protein is absolutely necessary to maintain life. In my life I have eaten every which way. When I was a self-proclaimed vegan, I took a deep dive into being a raw vegan. I found a class that looked interesting and my son, ten at the time, agreed to accompany me. It was a great class, and I learned recipes that I still use to this day. While we no longer follow that way of eating we both continue to love vegetables but now we add a healthy amount of protein to our meals as well. I also spent two years following a ketogenic diet. Although my lab work improved greatly from being off sugar and grains, my belly wasn't fond of the dairy. Over the years I have found a healthy balance of food choices that benefit me and my patients which has become The Supercharged Method.

We start with protein. Protein is important to repair and maintain muscle. Muscle is metabolically active tissue that allows us to get up from the floor, climb stairs, and for our heart to pump since our heart is also a muscle.

Dr. Daniel Amen, psychiatrist, brain disorder specialist, and director of Amen Clinics, and his wife Tana, a nutritionist, also promote protein (approximately 20 grams a meal) for overall health but especially brain health.

A serving size of proteins should be about the size of the palm of your hand, not including your fingers. This measurement works for chicken, steak, or fish and translates to about two to three eggs, one cup of beans or lentils, or a half a cup of dairy products. Ultimately a serving of protein should be 15–30 grams. There is about seven grams of protein in one ounce of cooked meat. An Example would be four ounces of raw, boneless, skinless chicken makes about three ounces of cooked chicken and provides 21 grams of protein.

Since height, weight, age, activity level and goals come into consideration when calculating the amount of protein recommended a day, it's easiest to use an online tool such as https://www.bodybuilding.com/fun/calpro.htm

People with kidney disease or those who are prone to kidney stones should consult their doctor for the amount of protein they should consume. You process protein through your kidneys, and if they aren't functioning properly it will put a greater strain on this vulnerable system.

PROTEIN POWDERS

You will get many more nutrients, release enzymes in the process of chewing and feel more satisfied if you eat food as

opposed to drinking it, but there are those times when a drink-
able meal is preferable. If you choose to drink a meal, choose
a protein powder that has no artificial sweeteners, chemicals,
or preservatives. If you are sensitive to dairy, do not use whey.
If you are sensitive to soy, do not use soy. There are a variety
of protein powders to choose from: rice, pea, egg white, bone
broth, grass-fed meat, whey, and soy. Choose one that has 15
to 20 grams of protein with under ten grams of carbohydrates.
Although gelatin and collagen are incomplete proteins because
they do not have all the essential amino acids, as long as they
are not your sole source of protein for the day you can include
those as well.

Protein	Serving size	Grams of protein	Calories
Almond butter	2 tbsp.	6	210
Almonds	1 oz.	6	165
Bacon	1 slice	3	43
Beans	½ cup	7	99
Beef (ground, cooked)	3 oz.	21	240
Beef (NY strip steak)	3 oz.	25	164
Cashews	1 oz. (15 nuts)	5	160
Chia seeds	2 tbsp.	5	120
Chicken	3 oz.	15	90
Cottage cheese (2%)	½ cup	13	90
Edamame	½ cup	11	120
Egg Whites	1 large egg	5	25
Eggs	1 large	7	80

Protein	Serving size	Grams of protein	Calories
Feta cheese	2 tbsp.	6	70
Fish (cod)	3 oz.	17	70
Fish (halibut)	3 oz.	19	94
Fish (salmon)	3 oz.	17	80
Fish (tuna, ahi)	3 oz.	26	110
Fish (tuna, skipjack)	4 oz.	25	110
Hemp seeds	3 tbsp.	10	180
Hummus	2 tbsp.	2	70
Lamb (chop)	3 oz.	12	170
Lamb (ground)	3 oz.	14	240
Lentils	½ cup	10	120
Peanut butter	2 tbsp.	8	190
Peanuts	2 tbsp.	7	160
Pine nuts	2 tbsp.	4	191
Pork chops	3 oz.	24	176
Pork (tenderloin)	3 oz.	22	125
Pumpkin seeds	2 tbsp.	6	112
Refried beans	½ cup	8	183
Ricotta cheese	½ cup	14	200
Shrimp	3 oz.	13	60
Sunflower seeds	2 tbsp.	3	102
Tempeh	3 oz.	17	163
Tofu	3 oz.	6	50
Turkey (breast)	3 oz.	26	125
Turkey (ground)	3 oz.	22	176
Whey protein powder	2 oz.	20	110
Yogurt (unsweetened greek)	½ cup	10	95

EAT TWO SERVINGS OF LOW GLYCEMIC VEGETABLES AT EVERY MEAL

A serving of low glycemic vegetables is half to one cup.

Low glycemic vegetables are less likely to spike your blood sugar (unlike corn, beets, or potatoes) when you eat them and contain essential nutrients and fiber.

THE GLYCEMIC INDEX (GI)

The glycemic index is a score used to evaluate to what extent a food raises blood sugar. The lower the glycemic index of the food, the slower it is released into the bloodstream. The more processed a food is, the higher the glycemic index, and the more fiber and fat in a food the lower the glycemic index. For example, commercial toaster pastries have a high glycemic index. Avocado has both fiber and fat which lowers its glycemic index.

Adding protein, fiber, and fat to a meal can decrease the glycemic index of the meal. This is one of the reasons that when creating a meal you should choose a serving of protein and two servings of vegetables (fiber) first, and then add a small amount of fruit or heavier carbohydrate source like a grain or potato to the meal with a healthy fat.

For example:

Broiled salmon (protein) + asparagus (vegetable) + roasted red pepper (vegetable) + half of a sweet potato (carbohydrate) with butter (fat) = a low glycemic meal.

The glycemic load is only slightly more effective in evaluating how a food affects blood sugar. So for the purposes of this book we will use the more widely referenced glycemic index.

- Low glycemic index (GI of 55 or less): All animal protein (chicken, seafood, beef), most fruit, vegetables, beans, dairy, nuts, and seeds.
- Moderate glycemic index (GI 56 to 69): White potatoes, sweet potatoes, corn, rice, and oatmeal.
- High glycemic index (GI of 70 or higher): Bread, crackers, cereal, cookies, and pastries.

Please do not obsess about the glycemic index. There is a reason I didn't include a chart of foods based on this system. The glycemic index of a food can vary based on how long it is cooked, how much it has been processed, the temperature of the food and when the food has been eaten in combination with other foods. That can get mighty confusing. Instead, enjoy your protein and vegetables. Avoid the pastries and prepackaged foods, and limit the sweet stuff, grains, and potatoes.

FIBER

Fiber has its own sordid controversy. We've been taught for many years that fiber is a necessary component to a healthy diet. That isn't true for everyone, and you need to find out what is right for you.

There are two kinds of fiber: soluble and insoluble. Most plants and grains (Fruits, vegetables, whole grains, and legumes) contain both. Soluble and insoluble fiber help maintain healthy blood sugar levels and insulin response.

Fiber keeps the bowel material moving in a manner that helps prevent constipation and diarrhea. Insoluble fiber, which does not dissolve in water, is the cellulose of plant material (roughage) and speeds fecal matter through the digestive tract, helping to prevent constipation by acting like a brush that moves fecal material through the intestines. Soluble fiber dissolves in water, creates a gel-like substance (think of how gooey oatmeal gets), slows digestion to possibly prevent diarrhea and potentially decreases cholesterol levels.

Fiber may alter your microbiome (the good bacteria that lives in your digestive tract). An article in *mSystems*, a journal through the American Society for Microbiology, documented a two-week study of increased fiber in healthy young adults. These individuals had increased their fiber intake from 15 grams a day to 40 grams a day, using mostly vegetables. This caused an increase in the beneficial gut bacteria bifidobacterium, bacteroides, and prevotella. These are species of bacteria known to break down fiber.

Some people who follow a lower carbohydrate diet for a variety of health issues will take fiber into account when they are counting carbs. "Net carbs" is the idea that since some fiber sources move through the intestines without being absorbed, there will be no blood sugar effect. For these people, who may try to keep their carbohydrate intake low (often to under 50 grams a day or less), every gram counts. Many manufacturers will add questionable "fiber" bulking agents in order to market their products to the population looking for lower "net carbs."

Here is an example: A small six-inch banana weighs approximately 100 grams. It has about 23 grams of carbohydrate and three grams of fiber. 23 grams of carbs minus three grams of fiber equals 20 net carbs. That is almost half of the amount of carbs allotted for the day for those counting net carbs. A half of an avocado is approximately 100 grams. It has approximately nine grams of carbohydrate and seven grams of fiber. That is a net carb count of only two. This is why those who watch their carbohydrate intake, and follow this idea of "net carbs," will include more avocado than banana in their diet. Oatmeal has 31 grams of carbohydrate and five grams of fiber in a half cup serving for a net carb of 26. You would think that oatmeal would have more fiber based on the advertisements. That's good marketing.

Some nutrition experts recommend that you get a whopping 30 grams of fiber a day. Avocados are not only a healthy fat source, but they are full of fiber. Brussels sprouts and cabbage are high in fiber, as well as most other vegetables and berries. Grains have their place here since this is a carbohydrate-conscious program, not necessarily a low-carbohydrate program, but the higher glycemic index of grains is why we limit them. I too would love to eat a loaf of bread a day, but that isn't going to help anybody's belly or blood sugar levels.

The Controversy

An interesting August 2007 article in the *World Journal of Gastroenterology* by Tan and Seow-Choen validates those who find they do not feel well from increased fiber. The researchers found that although fiber may reduce cholesterol absorption, it can also keep you from getting the nutrients (vitamins and the minerals zinc, calcium, magnesium, and iron) and enzymes needed to break down and digest your food, resulting in a decrease in nutrient availability. It can also cause fermentation in the gut and can lead to bloating, gas and, in some people, constipation. These are trademark symptoms of SIBO or small intestinal bacterial overgrowth that plague many with intestinal issues.

Vegetables are full of phytonutrients, vitamins, and minerals so make sure plenty of vegetables are included in your diet and keep the grains to a minimum.

Eat a wide variety of vegetables in a variety of colors. Think of eating a rainbow: red tomatoes, beets, and radishes; orange peppers, carrots, squash, and pumpkin; yellow summer squash and string beans; green spinach, kale, collard greens, green beans, and asparagus; and purple cabbage, onion, radish, and kohlrabi.

Try to include foods from these categories of vegetables each day:

- Anti-inflammatory and cell-protective cruciferous and sulfur-containing vegetables: onions, mushrooms, cabbage, broccoli, cauliflower, Brussels sprouts, asparagus, shallot, leeks, and garlic
- Gut healthy pre- and probiotic vegetables: fermented vegetables, sauerkraut, kimchi, pickles
- Nutrient-rich dark leafy greens: arugula, kale, spinach, swiss chard, collard greens, bok choy, mustard greens, dandelion greens, turnip greens, beet greens, watercress, broccoli rabe
- Iodine-rich seaweed and sea vegetables: kelp, dulse, kombu, nori, wakame, arame, spirulina, chlorella

The Supercharged Method
VISUAL GUIDE
to portion sizes

ONE PALM = ONE
SERVING OF PROTEIN

TWO FISTS =
TWO SERVINGS
OF VEGETABLES

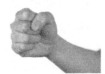

ONE THUMB =
ONE SERVING
OF FAT

ONE CUPPED HAND =
ONE SERVING OF
HIGHER GLYCEMIC
CARBS

ONE CUPPED
HAND = ONE
SERVING OF
FRUIT

Specific Wellness
clinics

EAT EVERY THREE TO FOUR HOURS

There is a ton of advice on what to eat and when to eat. If you found something that works for you that provides you energy, clarity, and focus, do that. If you didn't, read on. Food is fuel and if we keep that in mind, we can compare it to fueling your car with gas. When you want to get from one place to another you fill up your car with gas. You need enough to not get stranded on the highway and not so much that it overflows your tank and spills on the gas station pavement.

We want to eat enough to get us to ingest enough calories and nutrients to repair tissues, build and maintain muscle, support the immune and nervous systems, and provide us energy, clarity, and focus to get us to our next meal without burdening our digestive systems or storing it instead of using it.

Eating higher protein meals balances blood sugar and insulin better than high carbohydrate meals. Over the years I have been working with patients this method has worked the best: eating every three to four hours allows the digestive system to rest and digest between meals. It also allows blood sugar levels to fall which helps many of the body's processes. That means no grazing between meals. If you can get to the three or four hour mark hungry but not ravenous, you did a good job creating your last meal. You want to listen to your body and eat when you are hungry which is typically three to four hours after your last meal. If you are starving at the three-hour mark you could have used more protein, vegetables, or possibly even healthy fats at your last meal. If you are not even remotely hungry after four hours have gone by, you may have eaten too much at your last meal or are not in-tune with your hunger cues. Eating for fuel is important. You need to get those nutrients in to support a healthy body and brain.

A sample day may look like eating at:

7 a.m., 10 a.m., 1 p.m., 4 p.m. and 7 p.m. if you are hypoglycemic and do better eating every three hours.

It may also look like:

7 a.m., 11 a.m., 3 p.m. and 7 p.m. if you can control your blood sugar and not feel ravenous.

For those who are into intermittent fasting, or just are not hungry until later in the day, it may look like:

12 noon, 3:30 p.m., 7 p.m. In this case, I recommend three servings of vegetables at each meal in order to get more nutrients and increasing to 1.5 to two servings of protein per meal.

Some people who initially feel more comfortable eating every three hours may be able to slowly adapt to one of the other options over time. Do what works for you now because being consistent and integrating it into your lifestyle will give you the best results.

IN A 12-HOUR TIME FRAME

"The best of all medicines are resting and fasting."
–Benjamin Franklin

Your digestive system needs to rest. A minimum of 12 hours not only gives your digestive system a chance to complete digestion, it also allows it to rest. When you are snacking all day, you are using up a lot of energy and nutrients keeping your digestive tract busy. Your immune system is constantly on alert when you are eating. Everything you eat has to be broken down and evaluated by the cells of your intestinal lining before it gets to enter into your bloodstream. This is a main part of your immune system. When you hear on the news that a food item is being recalled, you hope your immune system is doing its job keeping whatever contaminant is present away from your bloodstream.

So, what is your body doing with all of the energy it's saving by not eating for 12 hours? The answer is repairing the tissues of the body and detoxifying or removing old, damaged and harmful cells.

You get to decide when that 12 hour fast starts. If you are a night owl and tend to eat late, you can implement strategies to extend your fast in the morning. Some strategies might be: staying busy, working out, or drinking water.

Stop eating three hours before bed.

You may notice you are more hungry in the morning if you have sugar before bed. Following The Supercharged Method should give you the nutrients you need to sleep well and wake up without being famished.

12 hours of eating, or less, and 12 hours of fasting, or more. Fasting has many health benefits, but you will have to experiment for yourself how much fasting is beneficial and at what point you are not getting enough nutrients throughout your eating period.

Benefits of a 12 hour fast:

Increased insulin sensitivity   Brain protective

Decreases inflammation   Increases Growth Hormone

Lowers LDLs and Triglycerides

As I was writing this book, my husband Tim reminded me of a time we were not on the same wavelength when it came to nutrition. It's a story he often tells new coworkers who proceed to tease him when he is hanging out by the vending machines. It was the early 2000s and the kids were old enough to watch movies at the movie theater. This was one of our favorite things to do and Tim would buy candy to eat during the movie. He was tired of spending four dollars a box so when Blockbuster (a movie rental place) offered ten boxes of candy for ten dollars he was overjoyed. He stashed those boxes of peanut M&Ms, Kit Kats, and Reese's Pieces in a pantry in our basement. The next time we were leaving for the movies he went downstairs to grab his favorite, Kit Kat. He noticed all the boxes were gone and in their place was an article on diabetes and the dangers of sugar, including pictures. I don't remember doing that but it clearly left a mark. His blood sugar is now stellar, by the way.

CHAPTER HIGHLIGHTS

★ Eating to balance blood sugar means low carbs and whole foods at meals without snacking.

★ Eat one serving of protein plus two servings of low glycemic vegetables every three to four hours in a 12 hour or less time frame.

★ You can add up to two fruits per day.

★ You can add up to two heavier carbohydrates a day.

★ Include four servings of healthy fats or oils a day.

★ No snacking between or after meals.

★ Protein is important to repair and maintain muscle.

★ Low glycemic vegetables are less likely to spike your blood sugar when you eat them and contain essential nutrients and fiber.

★ The glycemic index is a score used to evaluate to what extent a food raises blood sugar.

★ Adding protein, fiber, and fat to a meal can decrease the glycemic index of the meal.

★ Eating higher protein meals balances blood sugar and insulin better than high carbohydrate meals.

★ Eating every three to four hours allows the digestive system to rest and digest between meals. It also allows blood sugar levels to fall which helps many of the body's processes.

★ Your digestive system needs to rest; fasting 12–14 hours helps to do this.

CHAPTER 9

WAIT—THERE'S SOMETHING MISSING

When do I eat my fruit, butter, and potato? I know you are desperate to find out. Remember our first goal is to balance blood sugar. Fruit and higher glycemic carbohydrate foods affect insulin levels more than protein and low glycemic vegetables, so we want to limit those to balance blood sugar. On The Supercharged Method you are not avoiding carbohydrates, you are limiting them. There are plenty of choices when it comes to fruit, potatoes, rice, grains, and healthy fats, just in moderation.

YUMMY CARBS

Choose up to two servings of healthy higher glycemic carbohy-drates a day. That means you can throw a potato in with dinner or you can have rice with lunch. Or both. But remember these are foods that increase your blood sugar so make sure that you have them with the protein, vegetables, and fat of your choice so that you are not spiking insulin between meals.

Best Heavier Carb Choices:

- Potato
- Sweet potato
- Acorn squash
- Butternut squash
- Lentils (also a protein)
- Beans (also a protein)
- Rice
- Quinoa (also a protein)

NATURE'S CANDY

Add up to two servings of fruit a day, one serving preferably berries because they are high in fiber, low on the glycemic index, and high in antioxidants. That means you can have fruit with your sugar-free yogurt in the morning. Or you can make a shake with unsweetened yogurt, berries, and greens.

Remember that fruit alone is not recommended because, once again, it spikes blood sugar. Oh, and fruit juice is a hard "no." Fruit juice is fruit minus the fiber. The fiber is what slows down the load of sugar entering the bloodstream and the remaining sugary juice affects blood sugar that much more.

Be mindful of freeze-dried and dried fruit. The water has been removed so they are little concentrated packages of fruit. Think of the size of grapes versus raisins. A cup-full of grapes would be a thimble-full of raisins. Make sure to not overindulge. Beware of added sugar in dried fruit and a preservative called sulfur dioxide, not to be confused with the beneficial sulfur-rich foods like cauliflower and eggs.

THE HEALTHY FATS

Fat and oils do not spike blood sugar, but unless you are on a ketogenic diet, where fats are emphasized, they should be limited to one tablespoon a meal. One ounce of nuts or seeds, a quarter of an avocado or ten olives per serving because they are so calorie dense.

Healthy fats include:

Olive oil	Ghee	Olives
Coconut oil	Butter	Nuts
Avocado oil	Avocado	Seeds

Use olive oil for dressings or a low cooking temperature because it has a low smoke point.

Use coconut oil, avocado oil, or ghee (clarified butter) for higher cooking temperatures because they have a higher smoke point.

What is a smoke point?

I shared this before, but it's important to note. A smoke point is the point at which a heated oil goes from shimmering to smoking. This is when the oils break down and release free radicals which can lead to oxidative stress in the body. Free radicals can damage the tissues of the body, and oxidative stress can cause changes like making cholesterol sticky, leading to plaques that can cause a heart attack or stroke.

This is why you want to use a sturdier oil with a higher smoke point, like ghee, if you are frying or searing a steak. You can use medium smoke point oils for sauteing on medium heat like coconut oil or avocado oil. Save olive oil to use for dressings which do not need heat.

Include four tablespoons of really good fats a day in your diet. And some people should have even more. If you're inflamed you may need more healthy oils.

A large portion of your brain is made of fat, and eating healthy fats and oils helps protect your brain and will also protect your nervous system because your nerves are coated with a fatty sheath called myelin. Myelin is needed for nerve conduction. If you have any brain issues you want to have plenty of good healthy fats.

You want to avoid inflammatory omega-6 oils like canola oil, vegetable oil, or nut oils.

The Supercharged Method

Pick a Protein 1/meal	Pick 2 Veggies 2/meal	Pick 2 Fruit 2/day	Pick 2 Heavy Veg/Grain 2/day	Pick 1 Tablespoon fat or oil 1/meal
Beans	Artichokes	Apple	Beets	Avocado
Beef	Asparagus	Apricot	Carrots	Avocado oil
Bison	Bell Peppers	Banana (1/4 piece)	Parsnip	Butter
Cheese	Broccoli	Berries	Buckwheat	Coconut oil
Chicken	Brussels sprouts	Cantaloupe	Gluten-free oats	Flax oil
Chickpeas	Cabbage	Cherries	Potato (white, sweet, yams)	Ghee
Cornish hen	Carrots	Coconut	Quinoa	Lard
Eggs	Cauliflower	Fresh figs	Rice (basmati, brown, wild, jasmine)	Olive oil
Fish	Celery	Grapefruit	Split peas	Olives
Hummus	Cucumber	Grapes	Teff	Sesame oil
Lamb	Dark greens (spinach, bokchoy...)	Honeydew		Nuts
Lentils	Eggplant	Kiwi		Nut butter
Milk	Green Beans	Mango		Seeds
Peas	Lettuces	Nectarines		Seed butter
Quail	Mushrooms	Orange		
Shellfish	Okra	Papaya		
Tofu	Onion	Pear		
Turkey	Peas (snow, snap)	Persimmon		Nuts and seeds have minimal protein per serving size.
Venison	Pumpkin	Pineapple		Consider using them as fats
Yogurt	Radishes	Pomegranate seeds		unless you are
(Nuts)	Salsa (sugar free)	Tangerines		a vegetarian.
(Nut butter)	Sea vegetables	Watermelon		
(Seeds)	Squash			
(Seed Butter)	Tomatoes			
	Zucchini			

Balance your blood sugar

8 glasses of water a day

8 hours of sleep a night

20 minutes of self-care a day

Know your labs

Dr Stacey Francis

CHAPTER HIGHLIGHTS

★ Choose up to two servings of higher glycemic carbs a day.

★ Choose up to two servings of fruit a day (preferably berries).

★ Avoid eating any fruit between meals. No snacking.

★ Fruit juice is a hard "NO."

★ Choose one tablespoon of healthy fat per meal.

★ Nuts and seeds are a better choice for fat than protein.

★ Be mindful of an oil's smoke point.

★ An oil heated past its smoke point causes damage to the cells of the body.

★ Healthy fats are good for your brain and nervous system.

SECTION FIVE

CHILL OUT

"What if we recharged ourselves as often
as we did our phones?"

—Unknown

Did you know that zebras don't get ulcers? Robert M. Sapolsky wrote the book on it. He's a Stanford University biologist and he knows about the body's response to stress. Think about it this way. You are a zebra and you and all your zebra friends are hanging around the waterhole. Along comes a hungry lion. It looks like zebra is on the menu so you and your friends get stressed and scared. Your heart beats faster, your eyes dilate, and blood leaves your digestive system to supply oxygen and nutrients to your muscles because you and your friends need to run like...well, like a lion is chasing you because it is. You run like the dickens for all of 20 yards. The lion picks off the weakest or slowest zebra and just as suddenly as it started you can go back to chillin' because now the lion is busy chowing down on zebra meat and the zebra's not you. Stress for 20 seconds isn't giving anyone an ulcer.

You as a human on the other hand, are going to overthink everything, worry about everything, and ruminate about your decisions causing yourself a stress response that doesn't quit. This is called chronic stress and it's more dangerous than a McDonalds cheeseburger and a cigar combined. It is also another cause for severe fatigue.

CHAPTER 10

YOUR STRESS HORMONE PRODUCTION FACTORY— THE ADRENAL GLANDS

It all starts with your senses. When your senses alert you to danger, hormones get released from two glands in your back that ride on top of your kidneys called the adrenal glands. This can happen if you smell smoke, hear a gunshot, see a bear, taste something rotten, or even think something scary. These messages travel through your nervous system to your brain and your brain sends a signal to your adrenal glands to prepare to run or fight. This is where the term fight or flight comes from. From your adrenal glands stress hormones get transported through the bloodstream to their target organs. Your eyes will dilate so you can see more of your surroundings, the blood vessels to your digestive tract narrow (because digesting food is not important when you need to run for your life), oxygen-rich blood floods into your muscles, and your lungs increase their capacity to take in air. All of this to save your life or, if we are going to be less dramatic, take a kickboxing class from Hans. Your primitive brain really doesn't know the difference.

The adrenal gland has two areas where hormones are produced. The outer layer is called the cortex. This layer produces and releases the hormones aldosterone, cortisol, and dehydroepiandrosterone (DHEA). The inner layer is called the medulla. This layer produces and releases the hormones adrenaline (epinephrine) and noradrenaline (norepinephrine).

- Aldosterone: Regulates salt and water levels in the body which have an effect on blood pressure.
- Cortisol: Produced gradually throughout the day. Generated more in times of fight or flight (stress). Cortisol also has a downside due to it being hard to regulate. It can swing high or low contributing to weight issues, energy extremes and psychological imbalances. It can also induce insulin resistance.
- DHEA: Helps create the sex hormones estrogen and testosterone in both men and women.
- Adrenaline: A hormone and a neurotransmitter. Surges during fight or flight (stress), stimulating the sympathetic nervous system which speeds up heart rate, decreases sensitivity to pain, increases blood pressure, and opens up air passages. Increases blood glucose when the body experiences episodes of low blood sugar. This happens by releasing stored glucose (glucagon) from the liver.
- Noradrenaline: A hormone and a neurotransmitter that regulates the blood vessels and heart rate.

These hormones, when released at the appropriate time (but not for too long), help to keep the body beautifully balanced.

CHAPTER HIGHLIGHTS

★ Stress is protective.

★ Short term stress is helpful, not harmful.

★ Chronic stress is harmful.

★ Stress hormones are produced in the adrenal glands.

CHAPTER 11

CAUSES OF WACKY ADRENAL FUNCTION

As you go through your day there are three glands communicating with each other in response to stress. They are the hypothalamus, the pituitary gland, and the adrenal glands, and together they are called the HPA axis.

1. The hypothalamus gets input from the environment and the body to indicate when cortisol is needed.
2. The hypothalamus will then send a signal to the pituitary gland.
3. The pituitary gland releases a hormone called ACTH which stimulates the adrenal glands to produce cortisol.
4. Once there is enough cortisol in the bloodstream a signal is sent back to the hypothalamus to tell the pituitary to reduce production of ACTH. The adrenal glands, in turn, will discontinue releasing cortisol.

Since primitive times the body has been programmed to respond to acute stress. Alerted to danger, the body responds immediately and is able to either confront stress or flee from it.

Either way, the danger passes quickly and the body returns to a parasympathetic state of maintenance and relaxation.

Wacky adrenal function happens when this stress response is constantly stimulated by non-life-threatening situations leading to chronic stress.

This can happen from:

- Lack of sleep
- Stress (emotional, biochemical, physical, current and past trauma, hypervigilance)
- Illness
- Inflammation (from stubbing your toe to inflammatory bowel disease and everything in between)
- Blood sugar imbalance

A state of being in a depleted adrenal state increases stress which depletes adrenal function.

When this happens your body will be so busy making cortisol that it will not make enough of other needed hormones like progesterone, DHEA and testosterone. It will also use up vital nutrients such as B vitamins, magnesium, and electrolytes. Excess cortisol will increase inflammation in the body, contribute to diabetes and high blood pressure, and increase adiposity, also known as belly fat. Now I know I've got your attention.

CHAPTER HIGHLIGHTS

★ The HPA axis consists of the hypothalamus, pituitary, and adrenal glands.

★ The HPA axis communicates stress signals from the environment throughout the body.

★ When danger passes the body returns to a parasympathetic state.

★ Adrenal dysfunction occurs when the stress response is constantly stimulated by non-life threatening situations that lead to chronic stress.

CHAPTER 12

SYMPTOMS WHEN ADRENAL FUNCTION GOES SOUTH

Fatigue is the number one symptom of a damaged adrenal system but not everyone feels fatigue the same way. You don't have to be unable to get out of bed to feel fatigue.

Here are some symptoms of adrenal dysfunction:

- Difficulty staying on task
- Poor decision making
- Brain fog
- Poor memory
- Feeling tired even if you had adequate sleep
- Difficulty falling asleep or staying asleep
- Needing caffeine or sugar to function
- Needing alcohol or sleeping pills to get to sleep
- Salt or sweet cravings
- Feeling light headed when standing quickly
- Low blood pressure

- Overwhelmed feeling
- Difficulty exercising
- Low libido
- Easily irritable or agitated

As you can see, many of these symptoms look similar to the symptoms of hypothyroid, anemia, and blood sugar imbalance. That is why it is important to test.

CHAPTER HIGHLIGHTS

- ★ Adrenal dysfunction can look like other conditions.
- ★ It is important to test for adrenal function when symptoms are present.
- ★ Fatigue and brain fog are two of the many possible symptoms of adrenal stress.

CHAPTER 13

TESTING ADRENAL FUNCTION

Although salt cravings, irritability, and low blood pressure are common signs of poor adrenal function, there are two tests I want to cover.

Pupil Contraction Test

In a healthy state the pupils of our eyes will dilate or get larger in the dark to see better and contract or get smaller in the light. Remember when I told you how the pupils get larger during stress in order to see more of the danger around you? When you are in a constant state of stress your pupils have a hard time returning to a contracted state. These people will be extra sensitive to sunlight, preferring to wear sunglasses everywhere.

You can put yourself in a darkened room in front of a mirror and watch how your pupils react as you shine a light on your eyes. Make sure it isn't a strong light. You don't want to cause any damage. If your pupils are slow to respond you may have adrenal dysfunction.

Salivary Adrenal Stress Test

A healthy adrenal system releases cortisol in the morning. This allows us to wake up, get out of bed and be alert for the day. Here you would see a spike of cortisol detected in saliva. As the day goes on you would see less cortisol being released until it drops off. The low cortisol level at night allows us to settle down in anticipation of sleep. All this can be seen through samples of saliva that are taken throughout the day and then sent into a lab for evaluation.

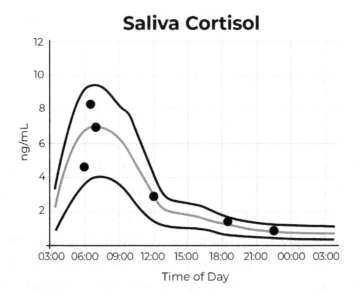

Notice these tests are not blood tests. No one wants to get poked multiple times in a day and since the cortisol levels move throughout the day we want to track its movement by taking multiple samples. So the best test for that is saliva. You spit in a vial at intervals throughout the day then send the samples to the lab for interpretation. The results will show cortisol levels that are reflective of adrenal gland function.

You might find you have low cortisol all day. Dragging yourself through the day with no energy. Another pattern might show that your levels are low in the morning making it hard to get out of bed and high in the evening making it difficult to get to sleep.

CHAPTER HIGHLIGHTS

★ Pupil reaction in the eyes showing a delayed response may correlate to altered adrenal function.

★ Cortisol levels can be tested by taking saliva samples throughout the day.

★ There is a pattern of cortisol levels that is considered optimal for most people.

★ Cortisol levels that don't fit the optimal pattern throughout the day may indicate altered adrenal function.

CHAPTER 14

SUPERCHARGE YOUR ADRENALS BY SLOWING DOWN

In many traditional medical settings the only adrenal conditions recognized are Addison's disease and Cushing's disease. Addison's disease is when the adrenal gland is damaged and can't function. Cushing's disease occurs when a tumor on the pituitary gland causes overproduction of ACTH and cortisol. It can also occur from the overuse of taking cortisol-like medication such as prednisone. These conditions should only be treated under the care of a trusted doctor. Functional health practitioners recognize that adrenal fatigue is a valid condition that needs attention and resolution.

Here are the many ways we go about repairing the adrenal glands.

1. Adequate sleep. This is why The Supercharged Method recommends eight hours of sleep and all the ways to get it. If you have adrenal fatigue you may need more sleep

than that. Take whatever amount of sleep that feels right to you knowing that you are helping to repair your adrenal glands. Include rest as well. This means you sit quietly, meditate, or deep breathe throughout the day.

2. Balance your blood sugar. That is at the core of The Supercharged Method. Blood sugar balance is necessary for energy, clarity, focus, and optimal health.

3. Reduce inflammation. Inflammation is behind every disease. Identify it and resolve it.

4. Chill out. Relax. Figure out how to do less. That might mean temporarily asking someone else to do more and that is okay. Recharge your batteries before it's a longer road back to recovery.

5. Mend your mindset. Be kind and loving to yourself and others. Trust that everything will work out. Stop watching the news with their shock and awe programming. Watch and listen to content that is nurturing and uplifting.

6. Seek therapy. Some specific techniques that help with stress, PTSD and other emotional dysfunction are Eye Movement Desensitization and Reprocessing (EMDR), Integral Eye Movement Therapy (IEMT), Neuro Modulation Technique (NMT), and Neuro Emotional technique (NET).

7. Rehydrate with electrolytes. There is a reason you crave salt when you are adrenal deficient. You have used up all your minerals and need to replenish them. Bone broth is one way to get important minerals; the other is consuming a half teaspoon of unrefined sea salt a day. I recommend Celtic Sea Salt and Redmond's Real Salt.

8. Adaptogens. I don't focus on supplements in this book but there are two supplements that I use with great success for energy and sleep in patients who are stressed. The first is called ashwagandha and it's an ayurvedic herb. It is called an adaptogen because it adapts to what the body needs. It can help you wake up in the morning and get to sleep at night. There are other adaptogens such as astragalus, reishi mushroom, licorice, schizandra, eleuthero, and ginseng. Find the one that works best for you.

9. B vitamins. This is the second supplement I use with my frazzled and fatigued patients. There is a reason why they are called stress vitamins. You use them up when you are under stress. Make sure to choose foods that are rich in B vitamins and consider supplementing with a complete methylated B vitamin complex.

Healing from adrenal fatigue takes time and patience. Don't give up and connect with a functional health practitioner if you need more support on this journey. 20 minutes of self care a day is the Supercharged way.

CHAPTER HIGHLIGHTS

★ Functional health practitioners recognize that adrenal fatigue is a valid condition that needs attention and resolution.

★ There are many ways to help the adrenal glands return to optimal function.

★ Resting the body and mind is often necessary to repair adrenal dysfunction.

★ The herb ashwagandha and the B vitamins, especially B12, are important nutrients that can help support the adrenal glands when the body and mind are stressed.

SECTION SIX

CHECK YOUR BLOOD WORK

"The goal is to turn data into information,
and information into insight."

—Carly Fiorina

I've lost count on how many times a patient thanked me for sitting down with them to explain the results of their blood work and how it relates to their symptoms. Everyone likes to solve a mystery, and what better mystery is there to solve than your own health puzzle?

CHAPTER 15

LABS, YOUR BEST FRIEND

This is the chewy section of this book. If you get anything from this section I hope it's that you can feel empowered by your health by identifying aspects that affect your health. You do not have to know how to read your blood work to get all the benefits of The Supercharged Method. You may skip the blood work altogether (especially if your eyes are glazing over from all the details) and utilize the recommendations in this book to get the energy you are looking for. If you haven't attained your goals, you can consider blood work at that time. You may also use this section to have a discussion with your doctor about your concerns and health goals. I hope you read this section and learn that you are in charge of your health and have access to information you may not have realized you could attain.

If you choose to do lab work, consider starting with a baseline and then do a follow-up three months after following The Supercharged Method. You will see your current status and then see what improvements you can achieve by following an enjoyable, sustainable and healthy lifestyle.

PROS AND CONS OF LAB TESTING

WHY YOU SHOULD DO YOUR OWN BLOOD TESTS

- You are your own best advocate.
- You can often use lifestyle changes to correct subclinical findings before they become clinical.
- You may choose to do labs that are not covered by insurance while your doctor needs an explanation to get approval from an insurance company.
- You want to be aware of your health risks.
- You may strengthen your relationship with your doctor.
- Some important tests are not routine and will not be done unless requested (such as vitamin D).

WHY YOU SHOULD NOT DO YOUR OWN BLOOD TESTS

- Having your doctor do testing allows for them to verify the findings and correlate them to the manifestations of the symptoms you are experiencing. Let your doc do what they were trained to do.
- Your relationship with your doctor. If you have a good relationship with them and they have your best interests at heart, they will not dissuade you from healthy diet and lifestyle changes to address a less than optimal state of being and resolve your symptoms of fatigue and brain fog.

- Overdiagnosis...you are not sick. Do not pigeon-hole yourself into identifying as being "sick." Your body is brilliant, and labs are just an indicator that you may have missed the mark on some aspect of keeping your body at an optimal functional state, sometimes through no fault of your own. (Hello genetics and environmental pollution.)

- Although rare, false positives and false negatives do occur. A false positive is a lab test that indicates that you have a condition that you actually do not have. A false negative is a negative result of a test for a condition that you actually do have.

- A marker out of range may be lab error. Sometimes checking twice is indicated.

- It may not mean what you think it means. Blood work is a guide and can be an indicator of a multitude of changes your body is going through. That is why periodic testing has value. Is the value moving more into range or out of range over time, and are there other factors related to that marker that are now showing up?

- The tests recommended for The Supercharged Method are directed toward information about blood sugar balance, anemias, thyroid function, and inflammation. If you choose to do genetic tests, tests for cancer, or tests for other life threatening diseases you should do them through your doctor. They will give you immediate support, a plan of action, and reassurance that you will not have if you choose to seek out these other tests yourself. Do yourself a favor, have back up.

REQUIREMENTS FOR DOING YOUR OWN BLOOD TESTS

- You are aware of false positives and false negatives.
- You are aware that results may be a lab error.
- You speak with your doctor about your goals and plans and get solid support.
- You educate yourself prior to getting your blood work.
- You are aware that medications and supplements can interfere with the test results.
- You are aware that the test results may be a result of recent dietary intake, stress, level of hydration, or working out.
- You are aware that whether Labcorp or Quest, you either need to stay with the same lab or start fresh with a particular lab and stick with it.
- You start comparing your results over time to see if there is a trend taking place.

This is why the method of this book is to fine tune your diet and acknowledge that exercise, sleep, relationships, stress, and the thoughts you think all have some weight in how you feel and how your body functions.

CHAPTER HIGHLIGHTS

- ★ Lab tests can be wrong.
- ★ Knowing your lab markers should only empower you.
- ★ There are pros and cons to doing your own lab work.

★ Being aware of your lab values can help you achieve your health goals.

★ You can be knowledgeable about your lab markers keeping in mind that no one marker stands alone.

★ Being under the care of a functional medicine doctor is optimal.

★ Always discuss out-of-range markers with a doctor trained in reading those markers.

CHAPTER 16

LAB RANGE VS. FUNCTIONAL RANGE

When looking at your labs there is lab range and functional lab range. If something is out of lab range, discuss it with your doctor—that is their domain and if there is something to do they will let you know. If it is out of functional range you want to do three things:

1. Make sure you are not taking medication, supplements, or anything else to cause it to be falsely out of range. The vitamin biotin is notorious for interfering with thyroid lab values.
2. Check the movement of the value compared to a previous test. Is it moving closer to the midline where it is a healthier indicator or further out of range?
3. Clean up your diet, hydration, sleep, and stress. In other words, follow The Supercharged Method for three months then recheck.

WHAT WILL THE BLOOD WORK SHOW?

When looking at blood work there are two main types of ranges:

1. A pathological range
2. A functional range

The pathological range is used to diagnose disease.

This is why your lab tests are "normal" but you still don't feel good:

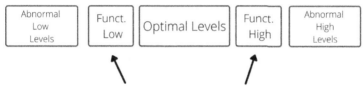

Functional ranges are the areas where you will find lab results that are considered "normal" but they are not optimal and you may still have symptoms.

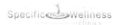

The functional range identifies risk for disease before the disease develops.

The references that are provided with laboratory test results are referred to as "the pathological range," because if the test results are out of range, it usually indicates **potential** for pathology or disease.

I have done my best to make reading blood work interesting. Think of it like a secret code that gives you the power to transform a simple message into information you can use to feel amazing. Isn't that powerful? It really is, and I can't wait for you to harness that power.

Data is wonderful. It can give you insight into what needs attention, and it can help guide your way. When I refer to lab work I am referring to the blood work that I recommend for The Supercharged Method and I will use the terms blood work and lab work to mean the same thing. Urine and saliva are lab markers, other than blood, that we also use to evaluate health. The lab work that I recommend are markers in your blood that can evaluate energy drains from blood sugar imbalance, iron transport issues, oxygen transport issues, and thyroid dysfunction. You can utilize the steps of this program even if you don't run your labs. If you choose to do The Supercharged Method without labs, you can skip this section and jump right into section seven.

If you don't already have blood work that has been taken in the last six months, you will want to order it. It may take a week or two to get the results, but don't let that stop you from starting The Supercharged Method. Having the blood work in hand will give you a complete picture of your health. Don't be intimidated. I am going to walk you through every step of the way.

We will be using the labs to guide us in what food groups to focus on to get the right nutrients. In most cases this is exactly what you need to get you to your goal of energy, clarity, and focus.

How To Read Your Blood Work

This is the part where I walk you through evaluating your blood work.

1. Print out your "MY LAB WORK WORKSHEET."
2. Pull up your most recent labs (within the last six months).
3. Fill out your worksheet by putting your lab values into the first column.
4. Notice on your blood work any H for high or L for low. Fill in an "H" or an "L" in the middle column where appropriate.
5. For the markers not marked with an H or an L, use the Lab Reference Page to evaluate if those markers are within or outside of the functional range. Use an "H" if it is above the functional range and an "L" if it is below the functional range, in the last column.

Look at your blood work.

Which, if any, markers have an H or L on the blood work, meaning they are outside of the lab range? If your trusted doctor did not already talk to you about these values, inquire.

If your values are within lab range, but out of functional range, The Supercharged Method is for you.

Action Tasks:

• Get blood work from your personal doctor or order online.
• Fill out the worksheet.
• Note if the values are outside of lab range, outside of functional lab range, or optimal.

LAB RANGES AND OPTIMAL FUNCTIONAL RANGES

BLOOD SUGAR MARKERS

	Quest Range	Labcorp Range	Optimal Functional Range
Glucose, serum, fasting	65–99 mg/dL	65–99 mg/dL	85–90 mg/dL
Insulin	</=19.6 uIU/mL	2.6–24.0 uIU/mL	<7 uIU/mL
HbA1c/Glycated Hemoglobin	<5.7%	4.8%–5.6%	4.5–5.3%
Triglycerides	<150 mg/dL	<150 mg/dL	50–75 mg/dL
Two hours postprandial glucose			<120 mg/dL

OXYGEN TRANSPORT MARKERS

	Quest Range	Labcorp Range	Functional Medicine Range
Ferritin	Men 19–59 Years 38–380 ng/mL >59 Years 24–380 ng/mL Female 19–40 Years 16–154 ng/mL 41–60 Years 16–232 ng/mL >60 Years 16–288 ng/mL	Male 30–400 ng/mL Female 15–150 ng/mL	Male 90–190 ng/mL Female 80–120 ng/mL

	Quest Range	Labcorp Range	Functional Medicine Range
Iron, Total	Men 20–29 yrs 50–195 mcg/dL >/= 30 yrs 50–180 mcg/dL Female 20–49 years 40–190 mcg/dL >/= 50 years 45–160 mcg/dL	Male >17 years 38–169 mcg/dL Female 18–60 years 27–159 mcg/dL >60 years 27–139 mcg/dL	50–100
TIBC	Male 250–425 mcg/dL Female 250–450 mcg/dL	250–450 mcg/dL	Male 250–425 mcg/dL Female 250–450 mcg/dL
MCV	90–98 fL	79–97 fL	82–89.9 fL
MCH	27–34 pg	26.6–33 pg	27–31.9 pg
Hb	Male 13.2–17.1 g/dL Female 11.7–15.5 g/dL	13.0–17.7 g/dL	Male 14.0–15.0 g/dL Female 13.5–14.5 g/dL
HCT	Male 38.5–50.0% Female 35.0–45.0%	37.5–51%	Male 40–48% Female 37–44%
Vit. B12	200–1100 pg/ml	232–1245 pg/mL	>600 pg/mL
MMA	87–318 nmol/L	0–378 nmol/L	<243 nmol/L

THYROID MARKERS

	Quest Range	Labcorp Range	Functional Medicine Range
TSH/Thy-rotropin	.40–4.50 mIU/L	.45–4.5 mIU/L	1.0–2.0 mIU/L
T4/Thyrox-ine, Total	Male 4.9–10.5 mcg/dL Female 5.1–11.9 mcg/dL	4.5–12.0 mcg/dL	6.0–12.5 mcg/dL
Free T4	.9–2.2 ng/dL	.83–1.77 ng/dL	1.0–1.95 ng/dL
T3/Triiodothy-ronine, Total	76–181 ng/dL	71–180 ng/dL	80–190 ng/dL
Free T3	2.3–4.2 pg/mL	2.0–4.4 pg/mL	2.4–5.5 pg/mL
reverse T3	8–25 ng/dL	9.2–24.1 mg/dL	10–15 mg/dL
TPO/Thyroid Peroxidase Antibodies	<9 IU/mL	0–34 IU/mL	<2 IU/mL
TgAb/Thy-roglobulin Antibodies	</=1 IU/mL	0–.9 IU/mL	<0.9 IU/mL

INFLAMMATION MARKERS

	Quest Range	Labcorp Range	Functional Medicine Range
hs-CRP	<1.0 mg/L	<1.0 mg/L	<1.0 mg/L
Fibrinogen	175–425 mg/dL	193–507 mg/dL	200–400 mg/dL
Sed Rate mm/hr	Male ≤50 yrs ≤15 >50 ≤20	Male <50 yrs 0–15 >50 yrs 0–30	Male <50 yrs 0–15 >50 yrs 0–20
	Female ≤50 yrs ≤20 >50 yrs ≤30	Female <50 yrs 0–32 >50 yrs 0–40	Female <50 yrs 0–20 >50 yrs 0–30
Homo-cysteine	Male <11.4 umol/L Female <10.4 umol/L	5.1–13.9 umol/L	<7.0 umol/L
25 OH Vit. D	30–100 ng/mL	30–100 ng/mL	50–90 ng/mL

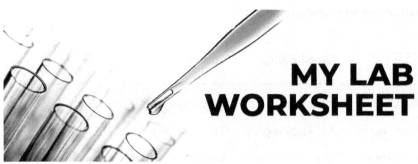

MY LAB WORKSHEET

	MY LAB VALUE	OUTSIDE LAB RANGE H/1	OUTSIDE FUNCTIONAL RANGE H/T
Glucose, serum, fasting			
Insulin			
HbAic/Glycated Hemoglobin			
Triglycerides			

Ferritin			
Iron, Total			
TIBC			
MCV			
MCH			
Hb			
HCT			
MMA			

TSH/Thyrotropin			
14/Thyroxine, Tota			
Free 14			
T3/Triiodothyronine, Total			
Free 13			
reverse 13			
TPO/Thyroid Peroxidase Antibodies			
TG/Thyroglobulin Antibodies			

-CRP			
Fibrinogen			
Sed Rate			
Homocysteine			
25 OH Vitamin D			

CHAPTER HIGHLIGHTS

★ The pathological range is used to diagnose disease.

★ The functional range identifies risk for disease before the disease develops.

CHAPTER 17

HOW TO PREPARE FOR THE BLOOD DRAW

Do not eat or drink coffee for 12 hours prior to the blood draw. This will ensure that you don't get a false high blood sugar marker. If you are pregnant or have other health conditions that require you to eat, consult your doctor first.

Do drink lots of water. You will have an easier time giving blood if you are well hydrated because your veins will be more accessible. Water is the only substance that will hydrate you sufficiently. Coffee can dehydrate you so stick with water.

I want to throw in this side note. Stress can affect your lab results.

In a December 2014 study in Health Psychology, 34 participants engaged in either stressful thoughts or distracted thoughts for five minutes at a time over a course of two hours. Their inflammatory and stress markers (C-reactive protein and cortisol) were assessed throughout the test. The group that ruminated on stressful thoughts had levels that increased and stayed increased after the exercise whereas the levels of the group that practiced distracted thoughts returned to pre-test levels.

Another study of 208 undergraduate students found that cortisol and cholesterol levels were elevated one to three hours before a major examination compared to three to four weeks prior to the exam.

Even a fight with your spouse or chronic psychological or social stress can cause enough change in your body to show on lab results. So thaw before you draw.

Do not use a single lone marker to determine if there is a problem. If multiple markers in any area (blood sugar, anemias, thyroid, or inflammation) are out of range, it bears attention.

Have each blood draw taken at the same time of the day for all follow-up testing. Values, such as iron, can drop throughout the day. You should not compare last year's iron value that was taken in the morning to this year's value that was taken in the evening.

Always use the same lab when comparing your lab work over time.

WHAT SUPPLEMENTS TO AVOID PRIOR TO YOUR BLOOD DRAW

Avoid the supplements biotin, iodine, tyrosine, and kelp at least three days before your blood draw since they can interfere with thyroid test results.

Avoid multivitamins, B vitamins, and iron two days prior, so as not to show a falsely elevated nutrient level that would hide an iron deficiency or B vitamin deficiency or anemia.

Do not go off any prescription medication unless your doctor recommends it.

WHERE TO GET YOUR BLOOD WORK

Most of the tests will be run yearly by your doctor, but there will be a few you will need to request or find on your own. You can also request the tests to be run through a variety of labs. Check your state to see which labs are available to you.

Other places to get blood work (at the time of this writing):

Walk-In Labs www.walkinlab.com

Direct Labs www.directlabs.com

Any Lab Test Now www.anylabtestnow.com

Life Extension www.lifeextension.com

LAB RANGES FROM LAB TO LAB

There is a range that labs use, and it differs from lab to lab. That means the lab Quest Diagnostics may have a different range than LabCorp.

	Quest Diagnostics Range	LabCorp Range
Insulin	</=19.6 uIU/mL	2.6–24.0 uIU/mL

When looking for trends over time, try to get your blood work through the same lab. The range these labs use is established after collecting data from a large population. Not necessarily a healthy population, just a large population. The optimal ranges are usually a tighter range that you want to be working toward. Don't get caught up in the numbers though. Watch the trend.

From the time of your last blood work to the next, you want to ask yourself, are you moving toward the optimal range? If you are, great. Keep doing that. If not, what can you do better? It is so important to watch the trend and not get caught up in any single number that happens to appear on an isolated day.

Lab errors happen more often than you think — approximately 12 million times a year, according to a 2014 study. Before you freak out over a lab result that is significantly out of range, get it tested again.

There is controversy regarding optimal ranges. People are all different shapes and sizes, they have different metabolisms and genetic abilities to perform functions such as detoxification. The reference ranges that conventional labs use do not account for those who are dealing with subclinical problems. The ranges I am using for "optimal" are the ones I use in my clinic after training with some of the brightest functional medicine and integrative doctors around. Lab ranges for a fasting insulin can range from <19.6 uIU/L for one lab to <25.0 uIU/L for another, but since insulin is only called out from the pancreas in the presence of carbohydrates (in most cases), insulin shouldn't even be roaming around the bloodstream if you have been fasting for 12 hours, so the functional range is much lower, but how low is debatable. I tend to prefer insulin levels under 11 uIU/L.

CHAPTER HIGHLIGHTS

- ★ Do not eat or drink coffee for 12 hours prior to your blood draw.
- ★ Be well hydrated with water prior to your blood draw.

★ Do not use a single lone marker to determine if there is a problem.

★ Have each blood draw taken at the same time of the day for all follow-up testing.

★ Always use the same lab when comparing your lab work over time.

★ Avoid taking multivitamins, B vitamins, iron, biotin, iodine, tyrosine, and kelp at least three days prior to your blood draw.

★ Do not go off any prescription medication unless your doctor recommends it.

★ The lab ranges for Quest Diagnostics and the ranges for LabCorp may differ.

★ Lab errors happen.

CHAPTER 18

EVALUATING BLOOD SUGAR IMBALANCE

Evaluating blood glucose, insulin, HbA1c, and triglycerides is important for more than identifying diabetes. If you are not managing your glucose and insulin metabolism you can face a multitude of other health conditions in the future. Kidney disease, liver disease, and heart disease can be repercussions from blood sugar imbalance as well as Alzheimer's and Parkinson's disease.

Keeping these levels in the optimal range will not only prevent disease but is the quickest route to regain the energy, clarity, and focus you are looking for.

GLUCOSE AND INSULIN

Fasting Glucose: Ideal 85–90 mg/dL

Fasting Insulin: Ideal <11 uIU/mL

Two hours after eating (postprandial) Glucose <120 mg/dL

I love talking about glucose and insulin. In my workshops you would see me making huge gestures with my arms to demonstrate how glucose and insulin work together to provide fuel to the body. It's a little more challenging to explain it on paper, so if I get a little elaborate and dramatic, brace yourself.

Let's start with the fact that you eat food because your body needs energy and you like food and don't want to feel hungry because that feels bad. So you eat, and depending on what you eat you will use one energy-replenishing system or another, a carbohydrate-based fuel source or a ketone-based fuel source.

A carbohydrate is anything that isn't fat or protein. All vegetables, fruit, grains, beans and legumes are carbohydrates. Protein is not a carbohydrate, but some protein becomes glucose in a process called gluconeogenesis. Even though it becomes glucose it doesn't raise blood sugar in most people the same way carbohydrates raise blood sugar. Certain carbohydrates release slower in your body than others. Refined carbohydrates, which are carbohydrates that have had the fiber removed, are quicker to absorb into your bloodstream. Think of whole grain bread versus white bread. It's white because all the fiber has been removed. The fiber needs more digestive time that, in turn, allows the carbohydrate to trickle into the bloodstream at a slower rate. This has also been referred to as slow carbs. Beans and lentils are slow carbs. When you eat refined carbohydrates with added sugar like cakes and cookies, or even in the form of sugar, like candy, there is no fiber to slow it down and it pours into the bloodstream from your intestines. When it crosses that intestinal lining and the carbohydrate enters the bloodstream, we now call that "blood sugar" or glucose. Glucose is necessary to use as a fuel source unless you are using another energy-replenishing system like ketones, but that is a subject we will save for another discussion.

Think of the bloodstream like a set of highways. You never want to just hang out on highways; it is just a quick means to get you to your destination. Glucose and insulin will be found in the bloodstream for an hour or so after you eat a meal with carbohydrates until they get to their destination. The destinations are red blood cells which bring oxygen to every tissue in the body, adipose tissue, which is the fat cells, the liver, the muscles, and the brain. Some of the glucose gets deposited into fat cells for storage. Insulin is like the key that opens the door of the cell to allow glucose to enter. Within two hours from the time glucose gains entry into the cell, there should be little glucose or insulin to be found in the bloodstream.

If left in the bloodstream, glucose can damage the inner walls of the blood vessel, causing nicks that contribute to inflammation and requiring LDLs to patch up damage in the vessels.

Let's talk a little more about how glucose enters the cell. Once the glucose gets to the cell you would think it could just enter the cell right there and then, but that is not the case. The glucose cannot enter the cell on its own; channels in the cell membrane need to open for it to enter. The presence of glucose signals a gland in your body called the pancreas to release the hormone insulin. It is insulin that has the ability to land on the cell and trigger a signal for glucose to enter the cell. Once glucose enters the cells, the blood sugar and insulin levels in your bloodstream drop. Mitochondria, the energy factory of the cell, uses the glucose to make energy. Now you have energy and feel full. Win!

There is a catch. When you overeat sweets or refined carbs you are at risk of overwhelming this system. An abundance of glucose in the bloodstream will trigger an overabundance of insulin to be released. Once this happens the vast amount of insulin will wear down the receptors on the cell membrane and signaling into the cell gets less effective. This decreases the body's ability to transport glucose into the cell. This occurs in brain cells as well. The cells remain energy starved without the glucose fuel that they rely on and you remain tired and hungry, and can't focus or think well. The insulin and glucose are just left hanging in the bloodstream where they are found when you get your blood drawn and we evaluate these markers. Excess insulin encourages more glucose to be stored in fat cells.

If you eat too many sweets too often, the insulin receptor sites wear down. Without adequate nutrients to build the receptors back up (Because how many nutrients are in a cupcake? Zilch!) you will find yourself insulin resistant.

Story time: It was 1992 and I was preparing to graduate chiropractic school. Knowing isn't doing, and although I knew not to eat all the crap I was feeding myself, I was under so much stress that I was making horrible food choices. The pressure of becoming a doctor and being responsible for the chiropractic care of my soon-to-be patients was overwhelming. The stress plus my poor eating choices made me terribly sick. I would grip the sides of my desk until my knuckles turned white just to bear the stomach pain I was experiencing and remain in class. I sought the help of a colleague who had recently graduated and practiced nutrition. She promised me she could help as long as I followed her instructions. The first thing she did was put me on a cleanse. No sugar, no flours, no processed foods, no caffeine, no alcohol, and no cheating. It was doable but not easy. I didn't realize how addicted I had become to sugar. It had become my escape, my comforter, my drug. Going off it was brutal. I remember finding a bag of stale christmas cookies in the closet of the chiropractic office I was working at. Not cookies I liked or would ever have chosen. An expiration date of more than two years old, they were just some long forgotten cookies that should have been thrown out eons ago. I honestly cannot remember If I ate them but I do remember the feeling of wanting to get that sugar hit again.

EFFECTS OF HIGH BLOOD SUGAR

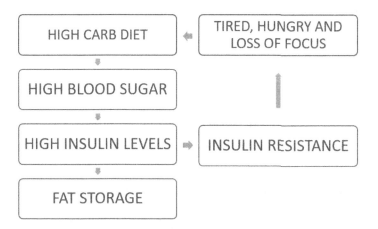

The Dangers of Insulin Resistance

- Poor energy production leading to fatigue
- Increased high-inflammatory belly fat
- Injury to the lining of the blood vessels
- Elevated inflammatory markers
- High blood pressure
- Decrease in growth hormone and thyroid hormone production
- High cholesterol

Another great test is a postprandial (after eating) glucose test. This test shows your body's response to carbohydrates. After you eat carbohydrates it takes some time to clear all the glucose in the bloodstream. By the two-hour mark, most if not all should be cleared and you should be back to your fasting blood glucose state. If you have a blood sugar device called a glucometer, you can perform this test in the comfort of your home. You can purchase glucometers online or at a drugstore.

Here is how to do it:

1. Eat a meal with approximately 75 grams of carbohydrates (a cup of rice and a medium apple is about 70 grams).
2. Wait two hours.
3. Take a glucose test using your glucometer.

   Results in the 80s are best, but 90–100 is also acceptable. If it is higher than that, your insulin receptor sites may not be sensitive enough to bind insulin to get glucose into the cells and out of the bloodstream.

A little side note about a ketogenic diet. Although lowering carbs can help with a multitude of ailments, a ketogenic diet is a significant decrease in carbs to the point that you are no longer using glucose for fuel. You have switched to using ketones for fuel. Many people thrive on this kind of diet, but not everyone. If you are doing a ketogenic diet without guidance you can easily either eat too few nutrients or deplete yourself of minerals and electrolytes causing fatigue, depression, and weight gain.

TYPE 1 DIABETES

Type 1 diabetes is an autoimmune condition where the immune system attacks the pancreas, preventing the production of insulin. It is usually diagnosed by the teenage years. Insulin must be injected into the bloodstream in order to be present to bind to the receptor sites on the target tissues.

TYPE 1.5 DIABETES

Also called LADA or latent autoimmune diabetes in adults, it may present itself like Type 2 diabetes but has the autoimmune component similar to Type 1. Addressing the autoimmune aspect of this disease using a focus on lifestyle is important and often helpful.

TYPE 2 DIABETES

Type 2 diabetes is when insulin resistance has gone too far and the insulin receptor sites are no longer sensitive to insulin. By following The Supercharged Method in this book you can balance your blood sugar to help prevent insulin resistance.

HEMOGLOBIN A1C

HbA1c Optimal Range: 4.5–5.3%

Hemoglobin A1c (HbA1c), also called glycated hemoglobin, is a blood cell that carries glucose around on its back for approximately 120 days. That means if you have had higher blood sugar because you are eating too many cookies and your body can't absorb the extra sugar into the cells, it's going to float around in the bloodstream. Since the sugar is sticky, it will attach itself to hemoglobin and float around for a while. When your blood is drawn, we can look at this particular hemoglobin and see that there is sugar stuck to it. So, this marker will show a kind of overview of your sugar levels over the last three months.

Things to keep in mind and why to not use a single lone marker as an evaluation of a condition: If you are anemic, have sickle cell disease, or have heavy periods, HbA1c can be falsely low. If you have iron deficiency or a recent blood transfusion, it can read falsely high.

TRIGLYCERIDES

Triglycerides Optimal Range: 50–75 mg/dL

Triglycerides are created to store calories that the body doesn't use right away. They are stored in your fat cells and are released for energy when needed. If you eat more calories than you burn on a regular basis, especially foods that are higher in carbohydrates, you may see that you have high triglycerides in your blood work. This is why high triglycerides may be a sign of blood sugar imbalance.

CASE STUDY

Jenny came to me after multiple attempts to lose weight and regain energy. Working on a construction site, she barely had time to breathe during her work week and made poor food choices when she was tired, bored, overwhelmed, or wanted to celebrate the weekend. (Does that sound like anyone you know?) Her labs came back and showed the following markers within lab range but out of functional range.

- ➢ Glucose 96 mg/dL (up from 92 three months prior)
- ➢ Insulin 19 uIU/mL (up from 17 three months prior)
- ➢ HbA1c 5.5% (same as three months prior)
- ➢ Triglycerides 100 mg/dL (up from 96 three months prior)

Looking at these lab values showed that, not only did she need more balance where her blood sugar was concerned, but that she was moving further out of range over time. Instead of beating her up and making her feel bad, we talked about where she was vulnerable when making food choices and how we could give her the tools she needed to improve her health.

Jenny noticed that when she was busy during her work day she often ignored her hunger cues and felt ravenous by the time she came home. That was when she ate her way through her kitchen until she was bloated and uncomfortable. She'd eat so fast that she didn't realize when she felt she had enough and only stopped when she was in pain from eating so much.

She agreed to take to work easy to eat, healthy snacks that she could keep in her jacket pocket. Beef jerky, kale chips, and sunflower seeds became her go-to meal when she didn't have time to stop for a meal. This allowed her to make better choices when she got home from work. The sweet tooth she had trouble controlling on the weekend was tempered by healthier low-sugar dessert choices. Many recipes she found were from wellness advocate Maria Emmerich.

In addition to the diet changes, I also recommended that she change some of her "stinkin' thinkin'" around her body image and her failed attempts at weight loss. I suggested she listen to podcasts by mindset authors and coaches Jon Acuff, Corinne Crabtree, and James Clear to start a better dialogue with herself.

In a short amount of time, Jenny regained her energy, lost weight, and balanced her blood sugar while eating meals she loved full of protein, vegetables, and healthy fats with occasional higher glycemic carbs like potatoes, rice, and fruit.

IF BLOOD SUGAR IMBALANCE IS INDICATED ON BLOOD WORK

One of the main keys to regain your energy, as laid out in this book, is to balance your blood sugar. The Supercharged Method is designed to help you do just that. One serving of protein plus two servings of vegetables, every three to four hours in a twelve hour or less time frame has helped thousands of my patients get back the energy they need to live a life they love.

I wish my family had practiced this method when I was growing up. My mom was notorious for making desserts. I remember as a kid she and my dad would have elaborate bar-beque dinners for their friends. The counter would be lined with layer cakes, colorful jello molds, and lemon meringue pies. What didn't get devoured that night would be put into the freezer for when guests came over. But it wasn't the guests that consumed those desserts. Late at night after my mother had gone to sleep, I would hear my father's footsteps in the kitchen. I would tiptoe down the staircase to find my dad pulling out the delectable frozen desserts. When he spied me, a huge grin would split his face. He and his partner in late-night-sugar-consumption crime would be at it again.

I cherish those memories, but as hard as my mother worked on those desserts, my entire family continues to work on controlling our sweet tooth and the fall-out from it. Follow Section Five to balance your blood sugar and move those less-than-ideal markers back into a healthy range.

BLOOD SUGAR AND YOUR BRAIN

To recap, you need the insulin signal to allow glucose into the cells. Eating too many carbohydrates causes the message into the cell to be diminished. When this happens you can't get glucose into the cell properly. This is called insulin resistance or impaired glucose metabolism. When this happens to the muscle cells your muscles become tired and weak. What do you think happens if this occurs in the brain?

Did you know that the hippocampus, the gland in the brain responsible for memory, has the same kind of insulin messaging needed to get glucose into the brain cells? This means that if the part of the brain responsible for memory can't get the fuel it depends on, it can become insulin resistant. When your memory center gets insulin resistant you can't fuel your brain, and dementia and Alzheimer's disease may develop. Alzheimer's disease is insulin resistance of the brain, or, as it's more recently been called, Type 3 diabetes. We all have moments of memory issues so don't run right out thinking you have dementia or Alzheimer's disease because you might be overwhelmed, tired, hungry, stressed, or a million other reasons, but keep in mind that bad habits that lead to insulin resistance can also have scary results.

OPTIMAL LAB VALUES FOR BLOOD SUGAR

Glucose, serum, fasting	85–90 mg/dL
Insulin	<7 uIU/mL
HbA1c/Glycated Hemoglobin	4.5–5.3%
Triglycerides	50–75 mg/dL
2 hrs Post prandial glucose	<120 mg/dL

CHAPTER HIGHLIGHTS

★ Evaluating blood glucose, insulin, HbA1c, and triglycerides is important for more than identifying diabetes.

★ Glucose is the most common energy source used.

★ Glucose comes from carbohydrates you eat which turn into blood sugar (glucose).

★ Insulin is needed to allow glucose into the cells where it can make energy.

★ Excess glucose gets stored as fat.

★ If glucose spends too much time in the blood vessels it can cause damage.

★ Excess insulin will wear down the receptors on the cell membranes and signaling into the cells gets less effective.

★ Excess insulin encourages glucose to be stored in fat cells.

★ Without adequate nutrients to build the receptors back up you will find yourself insulin resistant.

★ Hemoglobin A1c (HbA1c) is a blood cell that carries glucose around on its back for approximately 120 days.

★ Triglycerides are created to store calories that the body doesn't use right away.

★ If the part of the brain responsible for memory, the hippocampus, can't get the fuel it depends on, it can become insulin resistant and affect memory.

CHAPTER 19

EVALUATING OXYGEN TRANSPORT

Energy—or the ability to get your rear end off the couch, or run a marathon, or a million other actions including digesting your food and fighting off disease—requires oxygen.

If you lack enough healthy red blood cells to carry enough oxygen through your body to all the organs and tissues, you have anemia. Anemia is a main reason for feeling tired, looking pale, and being weak.

There isn't just one kind of anemia. There are several forms with many causes, and it can run from mild to severe. If your blood tests are outside of the lab range your doctor has likely already caught the anemia because it is one of the markers they look at on your yearly blood work. Suboptimal ranges can be just as debilitating as being out of range so we want to make sure that is identified and corrected.

Dr. David M. Goldstein, medical director of North Hills Natural Medicine LLC in Wexford, Pennsylvania, notes that conventional training teaches doctors only to recognize the most severe cases of iron deficiency, which is true anemia (low RBC count and low hematocrit). Anemia only occurs when stored iron (ferritin) is under the normal range. In holistic/functional medicine we recognize that you can be iron deficient WITHOUT being anemic. The need for iron is satisfied first by incorporating it into hemoglobin, but it has many more roles in the body that require higher ferritin levels. Iron is crucial to an optimally functioning body. For example, it is used as an essential substance in three separate steps in making energy (the Krebs cycle), as a cofactor for neurotransmitter production (dopamine and serotonin), as a central atom in the cytochromes used for detoxification in the liver, and it is used by white blood cells to generate free radicals to fight infection.

Iron deficiency is not the only deficiency that can impair oxygen transport. You can also have a folate or B12 deficiency. If we find it, we can correct it. We will cover that in the next chapter.

If you are within lab range but out of optimal range you could have poor oxygen transport and may be flirting with anemia. There are foods to include in your diet that can pull you back into optimal or functional range.

It is so much easier to identify imbalances early and correct them by improving your diet. If you wait too long you can develop a disease and need supplemental or medical intervention. We like to avoid medical intervention when possible.

There are many symptoms of poor oxygen transport, and they often overlap with other conditions. Do you have any of the symptoms below?

- Fatigue
- Feeling of unwellness

- Heart palpitations
- Hair loss
- Weakness
- Headache
- Pounding in your ears
- Brittle nails
- Pale skin
- Dizziness
- Rapid heartbeat
- Shortness of breath
- Cold intolerance / cold hands or cold feet
- ADHD
- Memory issues
- Nervousness
- Difficulty concentrating
- Postpartum depression
- Frequent infections
- Tongue swelling (sometimes indicated by teeth marks on the sides of the tongue)
- Irritation in the corners of the mouth (angular stomatitis)

If you do, let's figure out why and correct it.

We are about to get into the trenches of biochemistry, but I promise to make it as painless as possible. It's not brain surgery. I take that back, it kind of is, if we can call surgery correcting problems. We are certainly going to make the brain work better if we can give it enough oxygen.

Okay. Take a deep breath and let's go.

HEMOGLOBIN

Hemoglobin Optimal Range: 13.5–14.5 g/dL for women, 14–15 g/dL for men

Jerry was a new patient. Her main complaint was feeling tired with occasional dizziness. She had moved to Michigan from Montana and in all the chaos of moving, had not seen a doctor in a few years. As we talked, she mentioned that she often donated blood in the past but more recently she was turned away. That would have been a good time for Jerry to see a doctor. The preliminary test that blood donation centers perform when they take a sample from your finger or your ear is to make sure you have enough oxygen-carrying red blood cells to make it safe for you to give up around a pint of blood. Jerry was told at the blood bank that her hemoglobin was too low to donate blood that day. She forgot all about that conversation until we talked about it during her visit. Jerry did not know that her low hemoglobin and her fatigue and dizziness could be related.

Hemoglobin (Hgb or Hb) is the protein molecule in red blood cells that transports oxygen from your lungs to the rest of your body. It looks like a mess of curly ribbons.

Hemoglobin consists of:

- Globulin (a protein)
- Iron molecules containing a red-pigmented compound called heme

Hemoglobin contributes to the shape and red color of the red blood cell. If you don't have sufficient heme from hemoglobin, which is red, you will not have that rosy glow and may look pale. Abnormal hemoglobin contributes to the sickle shape of red blood cells in Sickle Cell Anemia.

If you have a darker skin tone you might notice that if you pull your lower eyelid down, the inside lid may look pale pink or yellow if you are deficient, instead of a bright reddish color if you have low hemoglobin.

One red blood cell contains millions of hemoglobin molecules.

I think of the red blood cell like my grandmother's purse that was filled with foil-wrapped Hershey's Kisses for when I was bored in synagogue. She would dole them out to me, and I would get an instant sugar rush and be happy as a clam... for about five minutes. There was always another Kiss in her bag. Those Kisses are hemoglobin, and her purse was the red blood cell.

Heme group chemical structure:

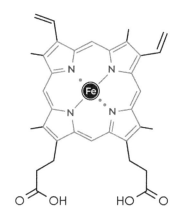

See the Fe in there? That is the abbreviation for iron.

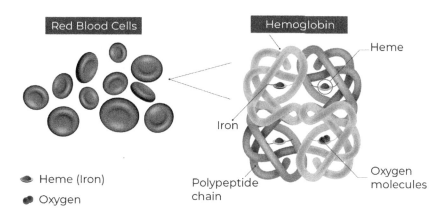

The hemoglobin count is an indirect measurement of the number of red blood cells in the body. This is why I didn't include a direct RBC level. It is typically included in the yearly blood work that your doctor performs.

When hemoglobin values are too low, it indicates anemia. Which is why we jumped right into talking about this blood marker. Anemia is a common reason for fatigue.

Symptoms of low hemoglobin:

- Fatigue
- Paleness
- Headaches
- Dizziness
- Lightheadedness

Causes for low hemoglobin:

- A lower level may be normal for that person
- Menstrual bleeding
- Pregnancy
- The body is producing fewer red blood cells
- The body is destroying red blood cells faster than it can replenish them
- Blood loss
- Certain medications
- Inflammatory bowel disease (ulcers, Crohn's disease, ulcerative colitis, polyps, hemorrhoids)
- Hypothyroidism (underactive thyroid)
- Certain diseases or conditions
- Iron deficiency
- Vitamin deficiency (B6, B12 or B9/folate)
- Smoking
- Dehydration

Usually, a high hemoglobin level does not cause symptoms, but can lead to complications that might affect the heart or lungs.

Causes for high hemoglobin:

- Polycythemia Vera (a bone marrow disease in which there are high levels of all blood cells)
- Heart or lung disease
- Liver or kidney disease
- Chronically low levels of oxygen
- Smoking
- Dehydration
- Any condition that contributes to a loss of fluids (ex: diarrhea)

In The Supercharged Method I will recommend nutrition that will support iron deficiency without anemia and other suboptimal conditions we will discuss.

If hemoglobin is low, we look at two other lab markers. One is mean corpuscular hemoglobin (MCH) and the other is mean corpuscular volume (MCV). This will give us a clue as to where the low hemoglobin could be coming from.

MEAN CORPUSCULAR HEMOGLOBIN

MCH Optimal Range: 27–31.9 pg

Mean corpuscular hemoglobin (MCH) refers to the average quantity of oxygen-carrying hemoglobin in a red blood cell. MCH levels are low in hypochromic (low pigmented) anemias which is any anemia where the red blood cells are paler than normal. It is calculated by dividing the total mass of hemoglobin by the number of red blood cells in a volume of blood.

MEAN CORPUSCULAR HEMOGLOBIN CONCENTRATION

MCHC Optimal Range: 32–34 g/dL

Mean corpuscular hemoglobin concentration (MCHC) represents the average amount of hemoglobin in a single red blood cell. MCHC takes into account the size of the red blood cell whereas MCH does not.

MEAN CORPUSCULAR VOLUME

MCV Optimal Range: 82–89.9 fL

Mean corpuscular volume (MCV) is the average size of the red blood cells. This plus a low hemoglobin level can be characterized into three conditions: overly big, or macrocytic anemia; too small, or microcytic anemia; and normal sized, or normocytic anemia.

Microcytic anemia is identified if hemoglobin is low and MCV is low and could be from iron deficiency (most common), chronic inflammatory disease, or thalassemia.

Thalassemia is an inherited disease where the body produces a low level of hemoglobin. Most people who have thalassemia get diagnosed as children. If hemoglobin and mean corpuscular volume (MCV) are out of lab range, bring it to the attention of your doctor so she can run a test for thalassemia.

Normocytic anemia is identified if hemoglobin is low and MCV is within range. Typically, the body cannot produce enough red blood cells. The size and hemoglobin content of the red blood cells are usually normal, but there are just not enough being produced. This is usually found in chronic infections and disease.

Macrocytic anemia is identified if hemoglobin is low and MCV is high. This can be from a vitamin B6, B12 or Folate (B9) deficiency, a low functioning thyroid, pregnancy, or drug/alcohol toxicity. Thyroid hormones play a role in the making of red blood cells, and iron. B vitamins are also needed for healthy red blood cells.

When a person has pernicious anemia, his or her immune system goes a little haywire and starts attacking itself, known as autoimmunity. When this happens, the immune system targets and destroys the cells of the stomach that produce intrinsic factor, a nutrient that must bind to B12 to be able to absorb. No intrinsic factor production means no B12 absorption, making you B12 deficient and anemic. In most cases, this will need medical intervention.

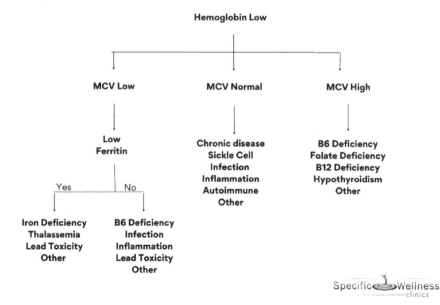

TOTAL IRON BINDING CAPACITY

Optimal TIBC Range:

250–425 mcg/dL for men

250–450 mcg/dL for women

Total iron-binding capacity (TIBC) measures the total amount of iron that can be bound by proteins in the blood. Since transferrin is the primary iron-binding protein, the total iron-binding capacity (TIBC) test is a good indirect measurement of transferrin availability—the amount of transferrin that is available to bind to iron.

HEMATOCRIT

Optimal HCT Range:

40–48% for men

37–44% for women

Hematocrit (HCT) levels show the amount of red blood cells you have in your body.

Whole blood is made of red blood cells, white blood cells, and platelets suspended in a solution called plasma. Your hematocrit level shows the percentage that is red blood cells.

CHAPTER HIGHLIGHTS

★ If you are within lab range but out of optimal range you could have poor oxygen transport and may be flirting with anemia.

★ Hemoglobin (Hgb or Hb) is the protein molecule in red blood cells that transports oxygen from your lungs to the rest of your body.

★ Hemoglobin consists of the protein, globulin, and iron molecules containing a red-pigmented compound called heme.

★ Mean corpuscular hemoglobin (MCH) refers to the average quantity of oxygen-carrying hemoglobin in a red blood cell.

★ Mean corpuscular hemoglobin concentration (MCHC) represents the average amount of hemoglobin in a single red blood cell.

★ Mean corpuscular volume (MCV) is the average size of the red blood cells.

★ Microcytic anemia is identified if hemoglobin is low and MCV is low.

★ Normocytic anemia is identified if hemoglobin is low and MCV is within range.

★ Macrocytic anemia is identified if hemoglobin is low and MCV is high.

★ Total iron-binding capacity (TIBC) measures the total amount of iron that can be bound by proteins in the blood.

★ Hematocrit (HCT) levels show the amount of red blood cells you have in your body.

CHAPTER 20

EVALUATING ENERGY PRODUCTION

B vitamins are essential for energy production. In order to make ATP, the energy "currency" our body uses for the numerous functions that keep us going, we need a healthy balance of B vitamins.

B-complex vitamins act as coenzymes in energy metabolism. Think of coenzymes as helper molecules. They are necessary in starting or causing a chemical reaction.

The B complex of vitamins includes:

- Thiamin (vitamin B1)
- Riboflavin (vitamin B2)
- Niacin (vitamin B3)
- Pantothenic Acid (vitamin B5)
- Pyridoxine (vitamin B6)
- Biotin (vitamin B7)
- Inositol (vitamin B8)
- Folate (vitamin B9)
- Para-aminobenzoic Acid (vitamin B10)
- Cobalamin (vitamin B12)

Although all of the B vitamins are important we will be focusing on vitamins B12 and folate.

COBALAMIN (VITAMIN B12)

Optimal Vitamin B12 Level:

>600 pg/mL

Cobalamin, also called B12, is one of the most important vitamins for energy production. It is also important for the brain, heart, and methylation (a process needed to keep us healthy).

When you are looking for energy, clarity, and focus, B12 is a rockstar. B12 helps produce red blood cells, and it helps release energy from food.

The sources of B12 are meat, eggs, and dairy. It is common for vegetarians and vegans to be deficient in B12 since the sources are mainly animal products. Those who choose these diets would benefit from taking a B complex supplement and B12 specifically.

Stomach function is important for getting adequate B12 levels. There are three compounds that must be present in your stomach for B12 absorption. They are hydrochloric acid (HCl), pepsin, and intrinsic factor. Hydrochloric acid, or stomach acid, and pepsin break down the cells that store the vitamin in order for B12 to be released from your food. Intrinsic factor escorts B12 from the food you are eating into the bloodstream. It is the bus that B12 rides on to go through the gut lining into the bloodstream where it can be used for energy.

As we age our ability to produce HCL decreases and this can lower B12 levels.

There is a simple test you can do at home to determine if you have sufficient stomach acid that we will cover later in this chapter.

Proton pump inhibitors, known as antacids, can also lower B12 levels since their purpose is to lower stomach acid. Since our digestive function becomes less efficient as we age, vitamin B12 becomes more difficult for our digestive systems to extract and from our foods and utilize. This is why the National Academy of Sciences recommends that anyone over the age of 50 take a supplement of vitamin B12 even if they eat meat.

Measuring B12 is not always accurate since its primary function occurs in the cell, not the bloodstream. When a B12 level is taken from blood work it indicates how much B12 is in the bloodstream, not the cells.

Some doctors think B12 is more adequately measured with a test called methylmalonic acid which we will talk about shortly.

If you are low in B12, you may have the following signs:

- Fatigue
- Brain fog
- Feeling depleted
- Moody
- Forgetful
- Light headed
- Tingling

If you are high in B12, you may still be low. B12 is carried in the bloodstream by two different transport molecules. They are called holoTCII and Haptocorrin, but for this purpose let's simplify it to carrier A and carrier B. Carrier A transports B12 through the small intestines, and carrier B transports B12 that has been stored in the liver. Although 80% of B12 that roams around in your bloodstream is transported by carrier B, it is carrier A that supplies B12 to the neurologic cells, which is very important for energy, clarity, memory, and stable moods. Some people who have low B12 from food intake or those on the medication Metformin may have low carrier A but normal or high carrier B (showing a normal or high B12 level in the blood). Thus your blood levels may be high but you might still be functionally deficient.

Keep in mind that the use of the medication Metformin is associated with B12 deficiency as shown in a May 2017 research paper in the *Journal of Family Medicine and Disease Prevention*. Researchers found at least 22% of Metformin users in that study had inadequate B12 status. In my own clinic, I notice that patients prescribed this medication are not having their B12 levels (or more preferably, their methylmalonic acid levels) checked routinely.

In fact, many people don't have their B12 levels checked enough. Take Jonah, a patient I see every month. He is a musician and a marathon runner. On one particular visit he told me about numbness he was getting on the left side of his face and arm. It was also on his left leg, calf, and foot. He noticed it at rest, while standing, and on and off while lying down. He was happy to tell me that it didn't get worse with running. It had started a couple weeks prior to his visit with me. We talked about his stress level, and although he had a lot going on and was busier than usual, he didn't feel particularly stressed. I adjusted the areas of his spine that showed imbalance that visit and saw him again after blood test results revealed he had a significant B12 and vitamin D deficiency. His symptoms resolved in a few weeks after supplementing appropriately.

What is important to note is that he isn't a vegetarian, so the deficiency wasn't from his diet, but he did have stress. He just wasn't aware that his stress was not due to emotional stress but from being so busy. How often are you so busy that you barely have time to sit down, or you say "I'm crazy busy"? This kind of busy stress, just like emotional stress, requires your body to utilize more B vitamins. It isn't that difficult to become deficient and get symptoms that will not resolve until the right test is performed and the correct action is taken.

METHYLMALONIC ACID

MMA Optimal Range: <243 nmol/L

There are two reactions in the body that need sufficient quantities of B12 to work. One is the conversion of Methylmalonic Acid (MMA) to Succinyl Coenzyme A which is necessary to make energy. The other is the conversion of homocysteine and folate to make methionine which is important for protein production, antioxidant production, energy production, and detoxification.

When you take Tylenol (acetaminophen), which is the most common cause of toxicity leading to liver transplantation worldwide, you can thank methionine for protecting your liver from acetaminophen poisoning.

Since vitamin B12 is necessary to convert Methylmalonic Acid (MMA) into Succinyl Coenzyme A, a lack of B12 will not allow the conversion to occur and MMA will build up in the blood. This is why a high level of MMA indicates a B12 deficiency.

This test is more sensitive than a straight B12 level in the blood. An October 2007 study in *Muscle & Nerve Journal* showed that a level of MMA higher than 243 nmol/L was a common finding in patients with polyneuropathy or damage to nerves that go to skin, muscles and organs. Symptoms may include burning, numbness, or tingling and may be improved with replenishing levels of B12.

Vitamin B12 is often deficient in vegan or vegetarian diets. Although nutritional yeast often contains vitamin B12 it rarely provides the amount that is needed if you follow a vegan or vegetarian diet. Supplemental vitamin B12 in the methylcobalamin or hydroxocobalamin form is recommended.

A methyl malonic acid (MMA) test, homocysteine level (which we will talk about later) and vitamin B12 level to evaluate vitamin B12 status will help you determine if low B12 levels are contributing to your fatigue and brain fog.

B12 SUPPLEMENTATION

Even if you do not have indications of a low vitamin B12 level, taking a trial of vitamin B12 is safe and effective. Vitamin B12 is water soluble and is eliminated easily. Even high levels have not been found to be problematic. If it feels good to you and helps improve your energy you can take it safely. Dr. David Brownstein's book *Vitamin B-12 for Health* covers this topic in great detail.

There are different forms of supplemental vitamin B12. Methylcobalamin, hydroxocobalamin and adenosylcobalamin are the preferred choices. Cyanocobalamin is synthetic and not as easily absorbed by the body. 1000 mcg of methylcobalamin daily is recommended.

Occasionally someone will have an allergy to vitamin B12. The reaction typically displays itself as an itchy rash that can have small clear blisters. This rash is similar to those seen with a nickel allergy. Nickel is a common skin allergen, often causing eczema. What do B12 and the mineral nickel have in common? B12, also known as cobalamin, has a molecule of cobalt in its center. Cobalt is next to nickel on the periodic table and can trigger the same kind of reaction in some people, especially if they have a nickel allergy.

Vitamin B12 is needed for every cell in the human body. Make sure this crucial nutrient is not overlooked when addressing your quest for energy, clarity, and focus.

FOLATE (VITAMIN B9)

Folate Optimal Range: 14–59 ng/mL

Folate is the natural form of folic acid. Folic acid is synthetic, or made in a lab, and is often found in fortified foods like cereal (Cheerios and Rice Krispies). Folate is essential for the body and works with vitamin B12 in many biochemical actions, like producing energy and detoxification. Folic acid, the synthetic form, can be harmful for some people.

A folate deficiency will cause the red blood cells to become similar to The Hulk—they become large and malformed. They can't function well in this new shape and tend to die off rapidly. We will talk more about folate in the inflammation section when we talk about homocysteine.

If B12 or folate are low, you are probably low in B6 as well. Although I did not include B6 in our lab panel, if you are interested in getting it tested, look for a serum pyridoxal phosphate test.

The nutrition recommended in The Supercharged Method focuses on B vitamins in addition to the nutrition needed to balance thyroid hormones, iron levels, and blood sugar.

IRON

Iron Optimal Range: 50–100 mcg/dL

According to the World Health Organization, iron deficiency is the most common nutritional deficiency in the world, followed by vitamin A deficiency and iodine deficiency. In the United States iron deficiency was second to vitamin B6 deficiency up until a few years ago. Currently Vitamin D deficiency tops the charts in the U.S.

Although low iron levels can mean a person is iron depleted it doesn't necessarily mean they are anemic unless hemoglobin is also low. Remember anemia doesn't necessarily mean low iron. It could also be low B vitamins, low thyroid, or other conditions or circumstances. If ferritin, which is stored iron, is less than 30 ng/mL, iron deficiency can be confirmed. Iron deficiency can also occur at much higher ferritin concentrations. More on ferritin shortly.

It is important to know how iron works in the body. Iron is necessary to transport oxygen throughout the body. B vitamins and other nutrients are also necessary to produce energy for the body.

Iron is needed for important cellular functions. It is needed for the brain to make the neurotransmitters serotonin and dopamine. It is also needed for white blood cells to make free radicals in order to fight infection.

Iron is a mineral that reminds me of Goldilocks and the three bears. Low iron will decrease the ability to transport oxygen for energy and too much will lead to oxidative stress causing damage to body tissues, DNA, body lipids, and the many other parts that make up your cells. Just like Goldilocks' porridge, chair, or bed, you want the amount of iron to be "just right."

Low iron is very common, and I encourage you to check it. Fatigue, weakness, and poor cognition (the mental action needed to think) as well as thyroid dysfunction are all associated with iron deficiency.

If you want healthy red blood cells you need iron. It is a trace element (you can find it on the periodic table) and an important nutrient. The body doesn't make it so it has to come from food or supplements. When you consume iron-rich foods, most of the iron forms proteins called hemoglobin which carries oxygen in red blood cells via transport with transferrin. Think of transferrin as the transporter of ferrum (the Latin name for iron). The rest gets stored as ferritin or used to make other proteins like myoglobin, which carries and stores oxygen in your muscles.

Because you can get too much as well as too little, iron supplements should only be taken when under the continual care of a doctor who is actively monitoring these levels. Some people have a genetic condition that causes the body to absorb too much iron, leading to higher than normal levels. This is called hemochromatosis.

Too much iron can be associated with heart disease, diabetes, Alzheimer's disease, and psychiatric disorders such as schizophrenia.

FERRITIN (STORED IRON)

Ferritin Optimal Range:

Female 80–120 ng/mL (menstruating and post menopausal)

Male 90–190 ng/mL

Iron is transported through the blood vessels bound to a protein carrier called transferrin. Transferrin will then release the iron it is carrying to the cells that need it. When the transferrin transport capacity is at its max (transferrin saturation), iron can circulate unbound or freely through the bloodstream. "Free" iron floating around in your bloodstream can damage cells. Your brilliant body will keep iron in a stored form called ferritin. When your ferritin level is low, it can be a way to detect iron deficiency at an early stage. When it is high, it can also indicate a chronic inflammatory condition. Since inflammation can increase ferritin levels, you may be iron deficient, but the inflammation is causing a false increase in your ferritin level. This is where you would look at other inflammatory markers of the body like C-Reactive Protein (CRP).

Ferritin can also increase with a higher body mass index and post menopause.

When ferritin levels are low but iron levels are within a healthy range, the stored iron is being used up even though there is still iron available to make red blood cells. It's just not being replaced in a timely manner. You may see a normal iron level and a low ferritin in this case. Once the stores have been depleted, you may experience an increase in transferrin and the binding of iron (total iron binding capacity or TIBC) as the body tries to mobilize more iron for the actions the body needs to function.

This is very important because fatigue and brain fog often result from depleted iron stores that could be found with a low (or even less than optimal) ferritin level, but not many doctors include it in their lab panel.

Remember, you can be iron deficient without being anemic. The many roles that iron has in the body require higher ferritin levels to accomplish them. Without enough iron, as indicated by a ferritin level of 80–120 ng/mL, you might find you don't have enough energy from lack of ATP, or feel depressed or anxious from a lack of dopamine and serotonin. You might also notice a higher sensitivity to toxins from an inability to detoxify adequately or a tendency towards frequent infections if you are lacking sufficient iron.

A June 2018 research article, published in the *Journal of Family Medicine and Disease Prevention*, demonstrates the importance of ferritin as a health indicator that can rule out iron deficiency without anemia. This article states that iron deficiency can account for 14–27% of doctors visits from women presenting with abnormal physical weakness or loss of energy.

Optimal levels for most people are usually 75–100 ng/mL. However, several studies show that 100–150 ng/mL would be preferable to prevent iron deficiency in individuals. A March 2018 study published in the *International Journal of Chronic*

Diseases indicates that a serum ferritin threshold of less than 100 ug/L or transferrin saturation rate of less than 20% can be considered diagnostic for iron deficiency in chronic disease of the heart, kidneys and bowel.

With hemochromatosis, a genetic condition that causes iron overload, it is best to keep ferritin under 50 ng/mL.

Iron deficiency and low ferritin can occur when:

1. There is not enough iron in the diet.
2. The body has difficulty absorbing iron from foods eaten or supplements taken.
3. There is a loss of blood.

Problems that Arise from a Lack of Iron

The body does not make its own iron. Iron has to come from the food we eat. Vegetarians, vegans, and those who don't consume iron-rich foods need to be aware of their iron levels and keep them in a healthy range. If this is you, get your ferritin level checked yearly and eat a diet that includes iron-containing legumes and vegetables. Eating them along with vitamin C-containing foods like kiwi, bell peppers, strawberries, citrus fruits, broccoli, tomato, and kale can help increase iron absorption.

Vegetarians and vegans should include the following iron-containing foods in their diet:

- Chickpeas, also called garbanzo beans
- Soy beans
- Lentils

- Black beans
- Pinto beans
- Green peas
- Lima beans
- Kidney beans
- Black-eyed peas
- Navy beans
- Northern beans
- Peanuts
- Broccoli

- String beans
- Swiss chard
- Beet greens
- Dandelion greens
- Collard greens
- Kale
- Spinach
- Cabbage
- Brussels sprouts
- Tomato

Poor Absorption

Those with celiac disease will have difficulty absorbing iron from their foods. Celiac disease causes damage in the small intestine when gluten-containing foods are eaten, causing the body to attack the lining of the small intestine. The small intestine is where iron is absorbed. The B vitamins folate (vitamin B9) and vitamin B12 are also absorbed here, and low levels of these vitamins can also cause fatigue.

Another example of poor absorption can be a lack of stomach acid. The ability to produce acid in the stomach decreases as we age. Stomach acid is needed to break down protein and iron-rich foods. When the body does not produce enough stomach acid your food does not break down enough to absorb the nutrients, like iron and B vitamins, and anemia can occur.

The Stomach Acid Dilemma

Correcting low stomach acid can be as simple as taking a supplement of apple cider vinegar capsules or betaine hydrochloride with meals, but don't run right out to get it before you read this. Low stomach acid can cause symptoms of heartburn and indigestion because the acidity of the stomach is what controls the valves at both the top of the stomach where the esophagus connects and the bottom of the stomach where the small intestine connects.

When it is time to eat, your hunger signals your stomach to start producing stomach acid. It continues to create stomach acid as you swallow your food and the food passes through your esophagus into your stomach. When the pH gets low enough from an adequate amount of stomach acid production it will signal the valve connecting to the esophagus to close. This is called the lower esophageal sphincter (LES). The LES stays open for a few seconds after you swallow. It closes to ensure that food and digestive enzymes don't flow up into your throat and stays closed the majority of the time.

Churning occurs in the stomach to break down the food you just ingested. Then the mix of broken-down food and acid passes through the bottom valve, called the pyloric sphincter, into the small intestine where you start absorbing the nutrients. If there is not enough stomach acid and the pH doesn't get low enough, the top valve, the LES, won't close adequately. The food and acid can then back up into the esophagus, causing heartburn and indigestion.

Taking over-the-counter acid blockers for heartburn will make the symptoms go away, but it won't resolve the problem. If the esophagus is already damaged from too much acid hitting the tissues, taking an acid supplement will be like pouring salt on a wound—painful. If you have reflux or indigestion, it may take some work to determine what is needed to resolve your symptoms and to correct the underlying problem but it is vitally important.

Symptoms of low stomach acid:

- Burping or bloating
- Gas after a meal
- Bad breath
- Constipation
- Sense of fullness during and after meals
- Difficulty digesting proteins and meats; undigested food found in stools

A quick test to determine stomach acid status:

Drink ¼ teaspoon of baking soda mixed with ½ cup of water on an empty stomach and use a timer to determine how long it takes to burp. If it takes more than five minutes to burp you probably have low stomach acid. Who doesn't love a kitchen science experiment?

If you have low stomach acid you can safely try taking capsules of apple cider vinegar with meals. If you have less gas, bloating, and burping you are on the right track. If it causes any discomfort, simply discontinue.

Pregnancy

Pregnancy can contribute to fatigue. When pregnant, the baby takes priority over the mom in obtaining nutrients like iron and B vitamins. If you are only consuming enough for the baby, you can develop anemia when the baby gets all the nutrients and there isn't enough left over for you. This can also be due to low stomach acid in the pregnant or nursing mom who may benefit from having this addressed.

Blood Loss

Crohn's and Colitis are other intestinal conditions that can cause blood loss due to inflammation and ulcers in the intestinal lining. The loss of blood can cause iron deficiency.

Have you ever had an ulcer? An ulcer occurs when the protective lining of your stomach, or the area of your intestines just past your stomach, thins. The acid of your stomach then damages the underlying layer, causing an open sore that is painful and can bleed.

Other than pain, symptoms of an ulcer can include bloating, burping, fatigue, weight loss, loss of appetite, black tarry stools, nausea, and vomiting. This can happen for a few reasons. Helicobacter Pylori is a bacteria known to contribute to stomach ulcers. Long-term use of nonsteroidal anti-inflammatory medication such as Aspirin, ibuprofen (Advil or Motrin), or naproxen sodium (Aleve) can also contribute to stomach ulcers. If you have an ulcer, stress and spicy food can make it worse. Have you ever had a cut on your hand and had to handle spicy peppers? The pain is severe, and the same thing happens when you eat spicy foods that flow over the open sore of an ulcer. Ouch.

Stress

Stress can also affect how your digestive system works and may even contribute to ulcers. Stress is when your senses tell your brain you are in danger. Like when you smell smoke, hear a siren, see an uncontrolled animal running toward you, or feel threatened in some way (like having a deadline that your job depends on). Under stress, your body switches from a state of "rest and digest" to "fight or flight." Rest means that you are in a state of low stress and digest means you are able to digest whatever food is in your digestive tract. This is the state that you are normally in when you are relaxed. It is called the parasympathetic state. The "fight or flight" state shuts off your digestive system (because digestion isn't essential when faced with a charging lion) and pools all your blood into your muscles to enable you to run fast or fight your way out of the situation. This state is called the sympathetic state.

When your digestive system is turned off due to stress, it stops producing the protective mucus layer. The acid that sits in your stomach, or just past the stomach, can cause irritation on that thin unprotected layer and can form an ulcer. This is how stress contributes to or aggravates an ulcer.

Because ulcers are an open wound they can bleed and often bleed a lot before you even know they exist. You might think you just have a common case of heartburn or indigestion. This internal bleeding can cause anemia.

Parasites

One of the more unique reasons for anemia, but still significant, is the presence of a parasite. Iron is a preferred source of food for parasites and other microorganisms. Parasites can impair your ability to utilize iron for your body's functions. Parasites can also damage the intestinal lining, causing irritation that may result in bleeding.

Menstruation

Women who bleed heavily during menstruation often have anemia. For some, monthly heavy bleeding during their period doesn't allow them to catch up on making and keeping iron reserves, and they may need to supplement or get injections of iron.

If you have been told you have low iron or anemia in the past, which might include being turned down to give blood at a donation center, or if your doctor has told you to take iron supplements then read the following section.

OTHER CAUSES OF LOW FERRITIN (STORED IRON)

- Medications
- Kidney disease
- Diverticulitis
- Autoimmune disease
- Sickle cell anemia
- Alcohol consumption

CHAPTER HIGHLIGHTS

★ B vitamins are essential for energy production.

★ Cobalamin, also called B12, is important for the brain, heart, energy production, digestive system, and methylation.

★ It is common for vegetarians and vegans to be deficient in B12 since the sources are mainly animal products.

★ Stomach function is important for getting adequate B12 levels.

★ hydrochloric acid, pepsin, and intrinsic factor must be present for B12 absorption.

★ As we age our ability to produce HCL decreases and this can lower B12 levels.

★ If you have high B12 levels, you may still be low in the actual amount of B12 available for cellular function.

★ Metformin is associated with B12 deficiency.

★ B12 levels and Methylmalonic Acid levels are used to evaluate B12 status.

★ Folate is essential for the body and works with vitamin B12 in many biochemical actions like producing energy and detoxification.

★ Iron is needed for the brain to make serotonin and dopamine. It is also needed for white blood cells to make free radicals in order to fight infection.

★ When your ferritin level is low, it can be a way to detect iron deficiency at an early stage.

★ Vitamin C and foods that are rich in vitamin C help with iron absorption.

★ When your digestive system is turned off due to stress, it stops producing the protective mucus layer.

CHAPTER 21

STEPS TO BETTER ENERGY AND OXYGEN TRANSPORT

It might take changing your diet altogether or just concentrating your choices on foods that will support your imbalances, but a diet change might be the only thing you need to change your energy status.

Absorption problems? Identify and correct them. Here is a clue. If you have had loose stools for a long period of time and you always thought that was just normal for you, try eliminating gluten for a few months. If it improves you may have the start of celiac disease or a non-celiac gluten sensitivity that can contribute to poor absorption. If you have symptoms of low stomach acid, take the baking soda test and try apple cider vinegar capsules.

Increased need? If you are pregnant and overly tired, because let's face it, creating a human is tiring work and requires more iron, then think about taking supplements. Get tested for what you are deficient in and at least take a prenatal multivitamin with methylated folate and Iron (as ferrous bisglycinate). Of course, consult with your doctor.

Blood loss? Sealing the leak is the first thing to do. If it is from a heavy period, balance your hormones. If it's from a GI bleed, have your doctor help you identify and heal. If it's from a parasite, let's identify that and eradicate it.

Not sure what to do? Always start with evaluating lab work to see if there is a deficiency.

High levels of ferritin can be due to:

- Inflammation
- Infection
- Disease
- Obesity
- Diabetes
- Fatty liver disease
- Alcohol abuse

CASE STUDY

Keira came to me when she was having difficulty concentrating at work as an engineer. I asked her about her energy levels, and she admitted that she would often rest her head on her desk for a quick nap during the day. I had her do a food log, and it showed that she ate a variety of vegetables throughout the day and a little bit of fish and tofu. We ran some blood work and it showed the following:

- Ferritin 32 ng/mL FL
- Total Iron 50 mcg/dL
- TIBC 320 mcg/dL

> ➢ MCV 81 fL FL
> ➢ MCH 30 pg
> ➢ Hb 13.2 g/dL FL
> ➢ Hct 39%
> ➢ MMA 92 nmol/L

All her lab results were within normal lab range which correlated to what her previous doctor found. Her ferritin (stored iron), mean corpuscular volume or MCV (the size of the cell) and hemoglobin (oxygen-carrying component) were all out of functional range. Compared to the previous labs that her doctor had run, she was trending toward a microcytic anemia, most likely from an iron deficiency since her diet did not contain a lot of iron-rich foods. She was willing to include some steak in her diet and even some chopped liver pate which she remembered her mom making when she was little. Within three months Keira's labs improved and it only took three weeks for her energy and focus to improve.

IF POOR OXYGEN TRANSPORT IS INDICATED ON BLOOD WORK

If your blood work indicates that you are not able to transport your oxygen adequately, due to any of the reasons we covered in the previous chapter, I am going to suggest you identify and correct any conditions causing it with your doctor. You should also eat foods rich in the key nutrients needed to support better oxygen transport.

As we just covered, "anemia" is defined as a low hemoglobin or low hematocrit. Ranges include Hb of less than 120 g/L in females and less than 140 g/L in males, but if you are borderline low or within lab range in these markers and the others we just covered, but not in optimal range, you may be headed for anemia. Why wait until your fatigue turns debilitating?

Remember to watch the trend and not focus on a single number. Be proactive with balanced food choices and work toward the healthiest body right now to avoid illness and live a life full of energy, clarity, and focus.

INCLUDE IRON-RICH FOODS

Iron is a mineral used in many biochemical processes in the body. It is needed to make thyroid hormones so you can regulate your body's temperature (so you're not so cold that you feel the need to dress up like the Michelin tire man in July) and metabolism (so you can fit into those jeans without lying on your back and sucking in your gut just to zip them up). You need iron to make stomach acid to digest that steak you ate last night. If you want to breathe you need iron. If you want that rosy glow so you don't look like Morticia Adams (my favorite Adam's Family character) then you need iron.

Before jumping into taking supplements, try getting iron from food first.

Eat liver

I can hear the "yuck" you just uttered. Liver is a superfood, and we don't utilize it enough. The benefits are plentiful. Besides a great source of iron, liver provides vitamin A, B12 and other B vitamins, minerals such as copper, zinc, and chromium, choline and coenzyme Q10. Hide it in meatballs or meatloaf if you have to.

Since the liver is a detox organ or filter, you want to get it from a healthy source that is grass-fed or you can get it from supplements.

Where you can find organic grass-fed liver:

- Farmers market (ask if it's grass-fed)
- Health food stores
- Heartstone Farm
- Grassland Beef
- White Oak Pastures
- 1915 Farm
- Starry Nights Farm
- Flying B Bar Ranch

When I was growing up, my mom would occasionally clear off our very cluttered phone stand and clamp an old fashioned meat grinder to it. I would watch as she ground up cooked liver and onions for a chopped liver appetizer she served on Jewish holidays. Growing up on the iron-rich delicacy, it brings back fond memories.

If you are not a chopped liver fan, hide it in chili. Soak a half pound of chicken livers in lemon juice and water for 12 hours. Saute with vegetables and process in a food processor before adding to a beef chili. It's undetectable.

Of course, there are sources other than liver. Grass-fed red meat, organ meat, clams, oysters, other shellfish, and sardines are great heme iron sources. Spinach, lentils, chickpeas, beans, tofu, chia seeds, pumpkin seeds and hemp seeds are all non-heme sources of iron. Some are better than others, but no matter which source you consume it's important to eat all sources of iron with a form of vitamin C, especially the non-heme sources. That means an iron-rich food eaten with broccoli, lemon or even lemon water will enhance the body's absorption of iron.

Conversely, calcium from supplements or cow's milk and milk products eaten within an hour of iron-rich foods or supplements can decrease iron absorption. So, avoid calcium and calcium foods an hour before and an hour after eating iron-rich foods if you are trying to absorb more iron.

Using a cast iron pan

If you are looking to raise your iron levels from using a cast iron pan, you might succeed, but it's hard to determine how much iron you are getting. Cooking food in a cast iron pan can raise hemoglobin, but the amount of iron you would get varies based on the acidity of the food, how long you cook it and the age of you and the cookware. When acidic liquids like orange juice are stored in a plastic container, the acid breaks down the plastic and pulls it into the juice. The same happens when you simmer tomato sauce in a cast iron pot. The acidic tomato sauce will pull iron into the sauce where cooking chicken in a cast iron pan will not draw as much.

A patient of mine will pull out her cast iron pan to use or will shelve it for a few months depending on her iron levels. This only works because she is consistently getting her iron levels checked.

THINGS TO BE AWARE OF WHEN INCREASING IRON

Constipation is a common side effect of increasing iron sources, especially iron supplements. Increasing fiber, magnesium, vitamin C, fermented foods, and prunes can all help relieve constipation. When choosing a supplemental form of iron, ferrous bisglycinate is more absorbable and stomach friendly than other supplement sources.

Not all iron sources are created equal. The iron that is consumed from animal sources such as red meat and liver is more easily absorbed than vegetable sources. This animal source of iron is called ferrous or divalent iron (Fe^{2+}) and can be stored as iron in the intestinal cells. The vegetable source of iron is called ferric or trivalent iron (Fe^{3+}) and in a healthy body, can be converted to Fe^{2+} in the presence of an acid, like vitamin C (ascorbic acid). Lastly, supplements can provide the body with the iron it needs.

Make sure to monitor your iron levels so you do not move too far in the opposite direction. You are already magnetic; you don't need to attract paper clips too.

INCLUDE B VITAMIN-RICH FOODS

There are many B vitamins, and they are all important but we want to make sure we get enough B6, B12, and Folate (B9). See the list below to know the foods to include to increase your B vitamin intake.

Remember the one serving of 15–20 grams of protein that goes with the two servings of vegetables I mentioned earlier in

Section Four? Well this is where you fine-tune your protein and vegetable choices to support your unique situation. If you are iron deficient you will add from the iron food list, and if you are B vitamin deficient you will add from the B vitamin food list.

Iron or B vitamin supplementation is necessary if you are significantly deficient or have difficulty absorbing your nutrients. You may even benefit more from iron IVs or B12 injections. Although B vitamins are safe to take, consult with your doctor if your markers are not improving with diet alone.

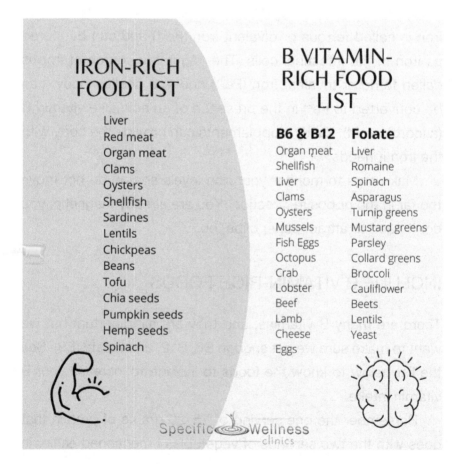

IRON-RICH FOOD LIST

Liver
Red meat
Organ meat
Clams
Oysters
Shellfish
Sardines
Lentils
Chickpeas
Beans
Tofu
Chia seeds
Pumpkin seeds
Hemp seeds
Spinach

B VITAMIN-RICH FOOD LIST

B6 & B12	Folate
Organ meat	Liver
Shellfish	Romaine
Liver	Spinach
Clams	Asparagus
Oysters	Turnip greens
Mussels	Mustard greens
Fish Eggs	Parsley
Octopus	Collard greens
Crab	Broccoli
Lobster	Cauliflower
Beef	Beets
Lamb	Lentils
Cheese	Yeast
Eggs	

Specific Wellness
clinics

OPTIMAL LAB VALUES FOR OXYGEN TRANSPORT

Ferritin	Male 90–190 ng/mL
	Female 80–120 ng/mL
Iron, Total	50–100
TIBC	Male 250–425 mcg/dL
	Female 250–450 mcg/dL
MCV	82–89.9 fL
MCH	27–31.9 pg
Hb	Male 14.0–15.0 g/dL
	Female 13.5–14.5 g/dL
HCT	Male 40–48%
	Female 37–44%
Vitamin B12	>600 pg/mL
MMA	<243 nmol/L

CHAPTER HIGHLIGHTS

★ Don't wait for a deficiency to eat foods rich in iron and B vitamins.

★ Liver is a great way to get iron in your diet.

★ Vitamin C helps absorb iron.

★ Poor digestive absorption can cause iron and B vitamin deficiencies.

CHAPTER 22

THE MIGHTY THYROID GLAND

The thyroid gland is a fascinating organ that resides in front of your neck. It produces the thyroid hormones Triiodothyronine (T3) and Thyroxine (T4). These hormones then get released into the bloodstream. The bloodstream is like a highway of vehicles that carry these hormones to every tissue in the body. Which means that every tissue in the body needs an adequate amount of thyroid hormones. Not too much, not too little, just that perfect balance. This provides your body with energy, a healthy thermostat, muscle strength, memory, and so much more.

Do you have symptoms of low thyroid? Check the following:

- Fatigue
- Brain fog
- Cold hands or feet
- Hair loss
- Low blood pressure
- Low body temperature
- Dizzy when you stand up quick
- Headaches
- Weight gain around your middle
- Loss of the outer ⅓ of your eyebrows

You might be wondering how your body knows when to make these hormones and how much to make.

Have you ever stepped out of your warm comfy bed, up to your ears in blankets, confronted with a very cold room?

Your temperature receptors in your skin will send a message to your brain to release a hormone called Thyroid Stimulating Hormone (TSH). TSH in turn will send a message to your thyroid gland to make thyroid hormones. With adequate hormone production, your body will kick up your metabolism, increase your heart rate and form "goose bumps" on your skin to heat up your body. This process and other internal and external stimuli

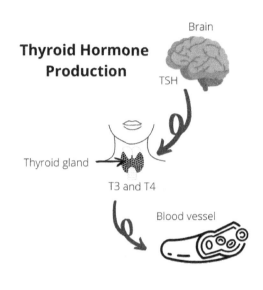

Thyroid Hormone Production

Brain

TSH

Thyroid gland

T3 and T4

Blood vessel

signal a message to your brain to "get the show on the road" when it comes to thyroid hormone production. Once you have enough thyroid hormones in your bloodstream the brain gets another signal to stop production.

Thyroid dysfunction is one of the more common reasons for fatigue and brain fog. Identifying and correcting a low functioning or an inflamed thyroid gland can prevent far reaching consequences because thyroid hormones are vitally important for every organ and tissue of the body.

Thyroid imbalance can contribute to the following conditions:

- Increased risk of heart disease
- Diabetes
- Dementia
- Memory loss
- Slow heart rate
- Rapid heart rate
- Low blood pressure
- High blood pressure
- High cholesterol
- Decreased ability to sweat
- Excessive sweating
- Kidney disease
- Fatty liver disease
- Obesity
- Vitamin D deficiency
- Osteoporosis
- Mood disorders
- And others

Symptoms of low functioning thyroid (hypothyroid: High TSH with Low T3/T4) include:

- Fatigue
- Brain fog
- Dry skin and hair
- Weight gain
- Cold intolerance

- Digestive issues like constipation
- Difficulty swallowing

Symptoms of overly high functioning thyroid (hyperthyroid: Low TSH with High T3/T4) include:

- Anxiety
- Feeling overheated
- Hair loss
- Weight loss
- Shaking or tremors
- Sweating

Thyroid hormones have many tasks. They help you burn calories, regulate your temperature and think clearly. Another task is to help make cholesterol and remove the cholesterol you do not need. This takes energy. Low thyroid function means you also have a lowered metabolism. Your thyroid hormones may be able to make cholesterol but may not be able to remove it at the required rate. When you can't remove LDL cholesterol efficiently, it can build up in the bloodstream. Even if your thyroid hormones (T3 and T4) are not low (I repeat—not low) a high TSH level alone can independently elevate cholesterol levels, as found in the August 2012 study published in *The Journal of Clinical Endocrinology & Metabolism.* When thyroid function is low, cholesterol levels rise. So, before agreeing to go on a statin drug to reduce LDL cholesterol, talk to your doctor about running a complete panel of thyroid tests to rule out a low functioning or inflamed thyroid gland.

HOW THYROID HORMONES ARE MADE

This lesson actually starts in your brain. You interpret signals from your sense of smell, taste, touch, sight and hearing and send messages to an area in the brain where two glands reside: the hypothalamus and the pituitary gland. As a result of specific messages, the hypothalamus will release a hormone called thyroid releasing hormone (TRH), not to be confused with TSH.

TRH will stimulate the front of the pituitary gland which in turn will release TSH, which we spoke of earlier in this chapter.

TSH, which is the most common test your doctor runs to evaluate your thyroid, will travel through the bloodstream and land on receptors on the surface of your thyroid gland. The thyroid gland sits in the front of your throat wrapped around your trachea or windpipe. As stated earlier, TSH will signal the thyroid gland to release thyroid hormones into your bloodstream. These hormones, thyroxine or T4 and triiodothyronine or T3, travel on a protein called thyroid binding protein through the bloodstream.

When enough of the thyroid hormones have been produced, a signal gets sent back to the brain to stop producing TRH and TSH to stop thyroid hormone production when there is enough. This is called negative feedback. "Negative" as in turning off.

When T3 and T4 get to the target tissue, which could be any tissue in the body because thyroid hormone affects so many areas, it simply jumps off the binding protein. Because it is fat soluble, which means it can go through fat, it will just shimmy right through the fat or lipid membrane into the cell. In the cell, T4 will convert to T3 because T3 is actually the active hormone, but because T3 can be toxic in high amounts, the body makes more of T4 and converts it to T3 as needed. T3 is what causes your metabolism to increase and stimulates your fight and flight system via the sympathetic nervous system response.

If you have low T4 you will most likely have low T3 because T4 is the main source of T3.

If you have difficulty converting T4 into T3 you could have a low T3 with a normal T4.

People with low thyroid function also have low metabolic rates. When you have a low metabolic rate you can't burn fat as easily so you may experience weight gain as a sign of hypothyroidism. A low metabolic rate can also make you tired, have cold hands and feet, and cause headaches and lightheadedness. On the other hand, people with high thyroid function, hyperthyroidism, or Grave's disease have an increased metabolism and increased fight or flight response. Here you might see a person who is losing weight, can't sleep, hyperactive, thirsty, sweats easily, and has a rapid heart rate. Hyperthyroidism can result from over medication, benign tumors on the anterior pituitary gland or thyroid gland, too much iodine intake, a goiter (enlargement of the thyroid gland), or an autoimmune disease.

AUTOIMMUNE THYROID CONDITIONS

Grave's disease is an autoimmune disease causing overproduction of thyroid hormone. Hashimoto's thyroiditis is an autoimmune disease that causes a fluctuating mess of both over and underproduction of thyroid hormone.

An autoimmune disease means that the body is producing a team of soldiers that mistakenly target and attack your own body tissue called autoantibodies. In Graves disease, the auto-antibodies target the receptors on the thyroid gland and act like thyroid stimulating hormone, creating a surge of thyroid hormone production. In this circumstance, the negative feedback doesn't work so the thyroid gland continues making thyroid hormones without stopping.

In Hashimoto's disease, the autoantibodies target thyroglobulin or thyroid peroxidase. Here the autoantibodies attack the tissue, causing destruction and inflammation of the thyroid gland.

WHAT CAUSES THE BODY TO PRODUCE AUTOANTIBODIES?

- Infection
- Toxins
- Allergic reactions
- Heavy metals
- Stress
- Inflammation

These can cause the body to get signals mixed and the immune system to target its own body tissue.

We can often reduce the intensity and frequency of the body attacking itself by decreasing inflammation using an anti-inflammatory protocol. We will cover inflammation later in this book.

CHAPTER HIGHLIGHTS

★ Every tissue in the body needs an adequate amount of thyroid hormones.

★ The thyroid gland produces thyroid hormones that provide the body with energy, a healthy thermostat, muscle strength, memory, and so much more.

★ Thyroid dysfunction is one of the more common reasons for fatigue and brain fog.

★ People with low thyroid function often have a low metabolic rate and experience weight gain.

★ A low metabolic rate can cause fatigue, cold hands and feet, and contribute to headaches and lightheadedness.

★ Grave's disease is an autoimmune disease causing overproduction of thyroid hormone.

★ Hashimoto's thyroiditis is an autoimmune disease that causes a fluctuating mess of both over and underproduction of thyroid hormone.

CHAPTER 23

EVALUATING THYROID FUNCTION

THYROID STIMULATING HORMONE

TSH Optimal Range: 1–2 mIU/L

Thyroid Stimulating Hormone (TSH) is released from the anterior pituitary gland in the brain to signal the thyroid gland to create the thyroid hormones Triiodothyronine (T3) and Thyroxine (T4).

In a healthy body, thyroid hormones stay pretty balanced. But when there are issues, TSH and thyroid hormones have an inverse relationship. For example, when TSH goes up too high, it causes the thyroid hormones to come down. Likewise when TSH decreases, it causes the thyroid hormones to rise.

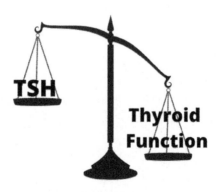

Low TSH can cause High T3 and T4 or hyperthyroidism (overactive thyroid function).

High TSH can cause Low T3 and T4 or hypothyroidism (underactive thyroid function).

Remember this when you are reading thyroid hormone levels. It can be confusing if you forget they have an inverse relationship.

The thyroid gland needs to be healthy in order to produce the right amount of T3 and T4. If it is diseased or damaged you might have a hard time producing enough thyroid hormones. When this happens it is called primary hypothyroidism.

The pituitary gland in the brain needs to be healthy in order to produce the right amount of TSH. If the pituitary or its neighbor the hypothalamus are diseased or damaged, you may not make enough TSH and also not get the signal you need to produce adequate thyroid hormones. You might have low TSH and low T3 or T4. Known as secondary hypothyroidism, this is less common and would require a consultation with your doctor.

Many doctors rely solely on the level of TSH to determine thyroid function or, at most, TSH and T4, but this is not a complete picture of thyroid function. Getting a full thyroid panel will help evaluate if nutrient support or antiinflammatory protocols may be needed to help restore energy, clarity, and focus and support the health of the thyroid gland before it becomes necessary for medical intervention.

TRIIODOTHYRONINE (T3)

Complete T3 Optimal Range: 80–190 ng/dL

Free T3 Optimal Range: 2.4–5.5 pg/mL

Triiodothyronine (T3) can be found moving through the bloodstream bound to a carrier protein. As hormones move through the body they have to be transported like cargo on a truck. Once they get to their destination they can detach from the carrier protein and attach to the target tissue like the heart or the lungs where they can affect the tissue. Unbound T3 is called free T3, and it is the most active of the thyroid hormones. "Active" means it can cause a greater response on the target tissue. The numeral "3" comes from the number of iodine molecules that make up this hormone—just as T4 is made up of four iodine molecules.

It is important to evaluate both free T3 and T4 as well as bound T3 and T4 (also called complete T3 and T4) in order to thoroughly evaluate thyroid function.

Being a more active molecule also makes free T3 more toxic in high doses. This is why the body, in its absolute brilliance, makes so much more T4 than T3. When needed, most bodies can easily remove an iodine molecule from T4 to create T3. Not every body can do this though. Some bodies have trouble converting T4 to T3.

If you have hypothyroidism you may be given a medication that consists only of T4. For those who need T4 and can convert it easily, this medication really helps. For those who have difficulty with this process, they need a product with both T3 and T4. This is where functional medicine practitioners really shine.

They can identify when you have a conversion problem and provide you with compounded thyroid extract or desiccated thyroid extract that has both T3 and T4 in just the right amounts for your body. They do this by paying attention to your symptoms and watching your blood work over time.

Yet we want to support the body naturally with the right nutrients before medication is needed. We do this by eating foods that are important for healthy thyroid hormone production and using supplements and medication if necessary.

THYROXINE (T4)

Complete T4 Optimal Range: 6–12.5 mcg/dL

Free T4 Optimal Range: 1–1.95 ng/dL

Thyroxine (T4) is an important thyroid marker to track from blood work. Low T4 will cause more TSH production. The rise in TSH signals the thyroid gland to make more T4 until no more is needed. A low T4 level can indicate hypothyroidism, and a high T4 can indicate hyperthyroidism. This can occur before the condition becomes so severe that T3 levels are even affected. Liver disease and medications, like lithium and some cancer drugs, can cause abnormal T3 and T4 levels.

REVERSE T3

Reverse T3 Optimal Range: 10–15 mg/dL

Another example of how brilliant the body is can be found here. Since too much T3 can be toxic, your body enacts a safety mechanism by converting excess T3 into a safe, inactive compound called reverse T3, also known as rT3, to get rid of the excess.

In some cases T4 will convert to reverse T3. When this happens, reverse T3, which is inactive, may bind to the same target organ sites that were meant for free T3. Leaving no room for free T3, which is active, can cause hypothyroid symptoms when the target tissue does not get what it needs to respond appropriately. This can happen from illness and increased levels of cortisol due to stress.

Starvation and illness increases rT3 and decreases T3. This makes sense since in a stressful state the body may protect itself by decreasing metabolism and conserving the energy that a high metabolism requires.

Stressful states benefit from more rest and a lower metabolism. Keep in mind this is any kind of stress, especially chronic low grade stress and post-traumatic stress disorder (PTSD).

Low iron levels, indicated by suboptimal ferritin levels, impair the ability to activate thyroid. This happens frequently in menstruating women. When this happens, rT3 is produced because these women cannot maintain a high metabolism.

We've talked about adrenal stress in a previous chapter, but it applies here too. Being in a depleted adrenal state increases stress. Increased stress contributes to thyroid dysfunction and adrenal dysfunction, which both can lead to increased stress. Do you see the vicious cycle?

If stress causes thyroid and adrenal dysfunction then we may also see an increased reverse T3 in cases of:

- Severe trauma
- Hypervigilance (a state of being highly or abnormally alert to potential danger or threat)
- Overreaction to stress (such as deadlines or an upcoming exam)

All of these can lead to an inappropriate fight or flight reaction.

THYROID PEROXIDASE ANTIBODY

TPO Optimal Range: <2 IU/mL

TPO is an enzyme found in the thyroid gland important for thyroid hormone production. An antibody is a protein in the bloodstream used by the immune system to identify and destroy anything that does not belong. Thyroid Peroxidase antibodies are specific antibodies that have targeted thyroid peroxidase for destruction.

TPO is high when the immune system attacks the thyroid gland and causes either high or, more commonly, low thyroid symptoms. This can indicate an autoimmune disease that targets the thyroid gland. In this case there is nothing wrong with the thyroid gland. The problem lies within the immune system which has been triggered to think the thyroid is a foreign invader and must be destroyed.

THYROGLOBULIN ANTIBODY

TgAb Optimal Range: <0.9 IU/mL

Thyroglobulin antibody (TgAb), which is part of the immune system, can cause an attack on the thyroglobulin molecule. Often removing gluten from your diet will help decrease this kind of attack for both TgAb and TPO because the molecular structure of gluten resembles the molecular structure of the thyroid gland. This is called molecular mimicry. If either of these antibodies are out of range, identifying the cause and decreasing inflammation in the body often relieves symptoms.

CASE STUDY

Cynthia came to me with fatigue. She told me that her mother and sister had been diagnosed with hypothyroidism, but despite having many of the symptoms, the blood work her doctor performed always came back normal. She told me she was always cold, her temperature ran low, and her blood pressure ran low. I could tell her hair was thinning, including the outer parts of her eyebrows. All symptoms of low thyroid. I could understand her concern. I asked her to bring in the blood work that was done to evaluate her thyroid function. She brought in four years worth from two different doctors. The only labs listed were thyroid stimulating hormone (TSH) and thyroxine (T4). I explained how the thyroid gland works and how there are many more components to thyroid function than she was having tested. She agreed to do more testing, and these were the results:

- ➢ TSH 3.8 mIU/L
- ➢ T4 7.0 mcg/dL
- ➢ Free T4 .9 ng/dL
- ➢ T3 90 ng/dL
- ➢ Free T3 2.2 pg/mL
- ➢ Reverse T3
- ➢ TPO 31 IU/mL
- ➢ TgAb .6 IU/mL

Looking at her results, we could see that not only was her thyroid functioning poorly, but it seemed the culprit was the antibodies (indicated by a functionally high TPO) that were attacking her thyroid. We discussed strategies to support her thyroid, decrease inflammation and avoid eating gluten. She was grateful we were able to get to the bottom of her symptoms, and she felt validated. It took some time, but she resolved most of her symptoms.

OPTIMAL LAB VALUES FOR THYROID MARKERS

TSH/Thyrotropin	1.0–2.0 mIU/L
T4/Thyroxine, Total	6.0–12.5 mcg/dL
Free T4	1.0–1.95 ng/dL
T3/Triiodothyronine, Total	80–190 ng/dL
Free T3	2.4–5.5 pg/mL
Reverse T3	10–15 mg/dL
TPO/Thyroid Peroxidase Antibodies	<2 IU/mL
TG/Thyroglobulin Antibodies	<0.9 IU/mL

CHAPTER HIGHLIGHTS

★ Thyroid Stimulating Hormone signals the thyroid gland to produce thyroid hormones.

★ Thyroid dysfunction is one of the more common reasons for fatigue and brain fog.

★ High TSH indicates a too low, or hypo functioning thyroid.

★ Low TSH indicates a too high, or hyper functioning thyroid.

★ A high TSH level alone can independently elevate cholesterol levels.

★ Unbound T3 is called free T3, and it is the most active of the thyroid hormones.

★ It is important to evaluate both free T3 and T4 as well as bound T3 and T4.

★ In some cases T4 will convert to reverse T3.

★ Thyroid Peroxidase antibodies are specific antibodies that have targeted thyroid peroxidase for destruction.

★ Often removing gluten from your diet will help decrease this kind of attack for both TgAb and TPO because the molecular structure of gluten resembles the molecular structure of the thyroid gland.

CHAPTER 24

IMPROVING THYROID FUNCTION

What are the treatments for hyperthyroidism, hypothyroidism, and autoimmunity of the thyroid?

The medical treatment for hyperthyroidism is to get the thyroid in a hypothyroid state. This is often accomplished by giving medication or radiation to stop the thyroid from overproducing thyroid hormone. This is always done under a doctor's care. A hyperthyroid condition should never be ignored.

The treatment for hypothyroidism is to get the thyroid to produce more thyroid hormone. In this case, the person is often given the oral medication levothyroxine or synthetic T4. In most people with hypothyroidism this works just fine because the person can convert the synthetic T4 to the active hormone, T3, in the body. Unfortunately some people cannot convert from synthetic T4 to T3 adequately. These people struggle the most with hypothyroidism. They ask, "Why isn't my thyroid medication working?" Oftentimes, these people lack the nutrients needed to convert appropriately and struggle with their hypothyroid symptoms like fatigue and brain fog in addition to weight gain, cold hands and feet, dry skin and hair, and lightheadedness. Selenium, iron, B vitamins, iron, and tyrosine will help combat these symptoms and are nutrients in the food you will consume if you follow The Supercharged Method.

The treatment of Hashimoto's and Grave's disease is an antiinflammatory protocol that will be covered shortly.

If you have been diagnosed with low thyroid and put on medication, you may still have fatigue and brain fog if the reason for the low thyroid function is autoimmune and isn't being addressed.

Has a family member ever been diagnosed with hypothyroidism? It can run in the family, so make sure to check your levels. Especially the autoimmune markers.

If you are on the medication lithium or the medication amiodarone, beware, because both can cause hypothyroidism.

Biotin use from supplements or multivitamins can result in falsely high T4 and T3 levels and falsely low TSH levels. This can lead to either an incorrect diagnosis of hyperthyroidism or that the dosage of thyroid hormone being given is too high. Always avoid biotin for at least three days prior to thyroid testing.

NUTRIENTS THAT SUPPORT THYROID FUNCTION

If you are within lab range but out of functional range, eating foods rich in iodine, tyrosine, selenium, iron, zinc, and B vitamins can help your thyroid function better by providing the nutrients that may have been lacking in your diet.

IODINE

Iodine is an important mineral, especially for your metabolism, because it is necessary for thyroid hormone production. Prior to the 1920's, the midwest region of the United States was known for its lack of iodine due to the effects of natural atmospheric processes. This area was labeled "the goiter belt" due to its high incidence of thyroid swelling from iodine deficient thyroid glands. Once identified by Michigan's Department of Health, iodine was added to salt to combat the issue. The rest of the country and then the world followed suit. By the 1950s, the observation of goiters in the midwest and then the world was greatly decreased.

Here is the catch. In the book, *Iodine: Why You Need It, Why You Can't Live Without It,* author Dr. David Brownstein states, "Although the addition of iodine to the salt supply has lessened the prevalence of goiter, it is inadequate to supply the body's need for iodine." Our bodies have a great need for iodine that iodized salt cannot fill. Not to mention the fact that salt has been vilified and blamed for hypertension leading to heart disease and stroke. The truth is you need salt (mineral-rich sea salt) as much as you need iodine.

If you are deficient in iodine you might experience your heart beating too fast or too slow; dry, flaky skin; tiredness; weakness; or feeling colder than you think you should or compared to the people around you. You might experience hair loss, a poor memory, difficulty learning, or weight gain. You may also notice swelling in your neck from a poor functioning thyroid gland.

Signs of Iodine deficiency:

- Fatigue
- Unexplained weight gain
- Carbohydrate cravings
- Hair loss
- Cold hands and feet
- Depressed mood
- Dry skin
- Brain fog
- Poor memory
- Goiter

Including iodine in your diet may alleviate these symptoms because it helps produce the thyroid hormones T4 and T3. Iodine helps remove toxins because it can bind to toxic metals like aluminum and mercury which you may have been exposed to from antiperspirants, aluminum cans or foil, or mercury fillings. It also protects the body from radiation poisoning. In fact, the U.S. military gives troops iodine supplements when they have been exposed to harmful radiation in the field.

Iodine is not just important for the thyroid. The whole body needs iodine. This important mineral helps with detoxification by flushing out other halides like toxic bromide. It helps clear mucus from the body's airways and protects mucous membranes. It supports breast tissue, and some doctors have found it is greatly effective in the treatment of fibrocystic breast disease.

Iodine rich foods (choose wild-caught):

- Kelp
- Seaweed
- Cod
- Tuna (choose wild-caught skipjack)
- Shrimp
- SMASH fish

What is SMASH fish?

Salmon, Mackerel, Anchovies, Sardines, and Herring make up the acronym, SMASH. They are the fish lowest in mercury and highest in nutrients like iodine, selenium, vitamin D, and anti-inflammatory omega-3 fatty acids that support the thyroid gland and immune system. Omega-3 fatty acids also reduce symptoms of cardiac and autoimmune conditions.

Mercury is a heavy metal that can cause neurological issues with overexposure in a system with poor detoxification.

Symptoms of mercury poisoning can be:

- Fatigue
- Anxiety
- Depression
- Brain fog
- Headache
- Memory loss
- Insomnia
- Gut issues
- Thyroid issues

Panic attacks; impaired vision, coordination and speech issues; muscle weakness; compulsive thinking; and sharp shooting pain in the body, including the face and head, can occur in severe situations. A study published in the journal *Biomolecules* in 2020 associated higher levels of mercury in the brains of patients with Alzheimer's disease. This is the reason that you want to avoid mercury whenever possible.

SMASH fish are typically easily digestible smaller fish with shorter life spans which translates to less time and space to accumulate mercury.

The daily iodine intake recommended is 50–200 mcg/day.

THE IODINE CONTROVERSY

Iodine is one of those minerals that, if you are old enough, you would know as the brown staining solution your mom would put on a skinned knee when you were young because of its amazing antimicrobial properties. Think of it like the Neosporin of its time. To this day it is still used as an antimicrobial in many doctor's offices. It is also one of the minerals located on the periodic table. Iodine is grouped with fluoride, bromide, and chloride because they are all halides. Halides are a group of minerals that compete for receptor sites in the body. Receptor sites are like landing zones on the surface of your cells that initiate a reaction. This is why, in the presence of excess fluoride, chloride, and bromide, you may find yourself deficient in iodine. You are exposed to fluoride in toothpaste and drinking water; chloride in cleaning solutions like bleach, city water, and swimming pools; and bromide from pesticide-contaminated flour used to make bread.

The most important job iodine has in the body is combining with the amino acid tyrosine to make thyroid hormone. This makes it an essential nutrient, and just like most nutrients, you must have the right amount.

Some practitioners think there is a significant deficiency of iodine in the food supply and in their patients, and these doctors have seen great, if not miraculous, results with including iodine supplementation in their programs. Other practitioners think there are negative side effects from taking too much iodine.

The truth always lies somewhere in between and is specific to each person. This is why The Supercharged Method supports iodine-rich foods. If you are interested in iodine supplementation, see a functional medicine practitioner you can trust to guide you in this manner.

TYROSINE

Tyrosine is an amino acid that helps the body build protein, formulate thyroid hormone, and produce enzymes and neurotransmitters. Iodine and tyrosine work together to form thyroid hormone.

Tyrosine-rich foods (choose organic, grass-fed, or wild-caught):

- Sesame seeds
- Chicken
- Eggs
- Cheese
- Turkey
- Soy
- Beef
- Lamb
- Fish

SELENIUM

Although it is used everywhere in the body, next to iodine, selenium is the second most important mineral for the thyroid. Selenium is used for every step of thyroid hormone production and function. This important mineral is also key in the production of the body's master antioxidant, glutathione. When glutathione is low or absent, free radicals can form that can damage the thyroid. Without selenium you cannot make glutathione, which can lead to thyroid disease and ultimately fatigue and brain fog.

When there is a deficiency of selenium, the thyroid has a hard time regulating iodine. Selenium allows for iodine levels to fluctuate without causing harm to the thyroid gland. Not only does selenium help in the regulation of iodine, but it can help prevent subclinical hypothyroidism, actual hypothyroidism, the autoimmune reaction to the thyroid and Hashimoto's disease. Have I convinced you to eat your Brazil nuts yet? It's important to get 100–200 micrograms of selenium a day.

In the case of Hashimoto's disease, selenium intake, via supplementation or dietary means, has been shown to decrease thyroid antibodies in three separate studies. It can even help prevent the eye pressure effect that people with severe Grave's disease (the most common cause of hyperthyroidism or overproduction of thyroid hormone) have, in addition to helping the thyroid heal from the attack of antibodies.

Brazil nuts are the best source for selenium. Eat 2–3 a day. If you eat more than four Brazil nuts a day watch for symptoms of overconsumption of selenium which can cause diarrhea and joint pain. Other sources include organic, wild-caught, or grass-fed:

- S.M.A.S.H fish
- Tuna (choose skipjack)
- Cod
- Shrimp
- Halibut
- Scallops
- Shiitake and crimini mushrooms
- Chicken
- Lamb
- Turkey
- Eggs

Sunflower seeds and brown rice are also sources of selenium but not as great as Brazil nuts.

Brazil nuts, which are actually seeds about the size of your thumb, are a powerhouse of nutrients. They are one of the best sources of selenium with 70–90 micrograms per nut. Calcium, magnesium, and potassium, in addition to zinc, iron, and phosphorus give this nut plenty of antioxidant and anti-inflammatory properties.

According to a study in the *European Journal of Nutrition* and an article in the publication *Biological Trace Element Research*:

- One single Brazil nut a day has been shown to decrease inflammation and signs of damage to cellular tissue called oxidative stress.
- The amount of selenium in one single Brazil nut can help optimize selenium levels that will support thyroid function and help convert the thyroid hormone thyroxine (T4) to the active hormone triiodothyronine (T3).
- One single Brazil nut for eight weeks has the ability to decrease total cholesterol and fasting blood sugar levels.

IRON

We covered the importance of iron previously. In addition to iodine, tyrosine, selenium, and zinc, iron is needed to convert thyroid hormone T4 to T3.

Iron-rich foods (choose organic, grass-fed, or wild-caught):

- Liver
- Beef
- Chicken
- Shellfish
- Sardines
- Beans

ZINC

Zinc is a mineral that, when deficient, can contribute to fatigue. It is essential for your body to produce energy. Zinc deficiency can be indicated if alkaline phosphatase, a marker often drawn for blood work, is at a level below 70 IU/L.

Zinc-rich foods (choose organic, grass-fed, or wild-caught):

- Lamb
- Pumpkin seeds
- Oysters
- Grass-fed beef
- Chickpeas
- Cocoa powder
- Cashews
- Mushrooms
- Spinach

Make sure these foods are included in your food choices throughout the week to ensure all the necessary nutrients for thyroid health are present. If you are low in these nutrients, your thyroid cannot adequately produce hormones, convert T4 to T3, or get T3 into your cells to attach to thyroid receptors, which can cause hypothyroidism symptoms, such as thyroid-related hair loss. I recommend a diet with plenty of organic, grass-fed, pasture-raised proteins, leafy greens, vegetables, organic fruits and healthy fats.

FOODS TO SUPPORT THYROID FUNCTION

SELENIUM	IODINE	ZINC	RIBOFLAVIN
Brazil Nuts	Kelp	Lamb	Eggs
Salmon	Seaweed	Pumpkin	Liver
Mackerel	Cod	seeds	Asparagus
Anchovies	Tuna	Oysters	Broccoli
Sardines	Shrimp	Grass-fed beef	Spinach
Halibut	Salmon	Chickpeas	
Tuna	Mackerel	Cocoa	
Cod	Anchovies	Cashews	**NIACIN**
Shrimp	Sardines	Mushrooms	Fish
Scallops	Halibut	Spinach	Liver
Chicken			Beef
Lamb			Turkey
Turkey			Chicken
Eggs			
Shitake & Crimini Mushrooms			
Sunflower Seeds			
Brown Rice			

Specific Wellness
clinics

CHAPTER HIGHLIGHTS

★ Hyperthyroidism is treated by inducing a hypothyroid state.

★ Hypothyroidism is treated by increasing thyroid hormone production.

★ Hashimoto's disease and Graves disease are autoimmune conditions.

★ Some people cannot convert from synthetic T4 to T3 adequately.

★ Biotin needs to be avoided for three days before thyroid lab tests are run.

★ Iodine is an important mineral, especially for your metabolism, because it is necessary for thyroid hormone production.

★ Tyrosine is an amino acid that helps the body build protein, formulate thyroid hormone, and produce enzymes and neurotransmitters.

★ Selenium helps in the production of glutathione. When glutathione is low or absent, free radicals can form that can damage the thyroid.

★ Iron is needed to convert thyroid hormone T4 to T3.

★ Zinc is essential for the body to produce energy.

CHAPTER 25

EVALUATING INFLAMMATION

Inflammation is your body's way of protecting you. A fever is inflammation, and it helps you fight infection. When you bruise you create inflammation, and it helps your body tissues go through a healing process. This is all good and appropriate inflammation, and we are lucky to have it.

When inflammation occurs throughout the body (systemic) over a long period of time (chronic), it becomes a risk factor for many disease processes. Think of it like a runaway brush fire. You need to know it's there to tame it, but if you wait too long it's difficult to contain. That is why it is so important to have these tests done routinely and practice lifestyle changes to correct inflammation before it creates a chronic, serious condition.

Inflammation can be associated with:

Autoimmune Disease Fatty Liver Disease

Diabetes Heart Disease

Insulin Resistance Heart Failure

Hardening of the Arteries   Dementia

Infection   Alzheimer's Disease

Injury   Osteoporosis

Stroke

There are inflammatory tests that can indicate that inflammation is occurring in the body.

High Sensitivity C-Reactive Protein or hs-CRP

Optimal levels <1 mg/L

This is a compound released from the liver when inflammation is present. It is not specific but it is sensitive and can indicate inflammation if you have heart disease or bumped your elbow. It can indicate acute inflammation such as a recent flare of arthritis, a tooth infection, or episode of inflammatory bowel disease. It can also indicate chronic inflammation. A 2018 study in *Frontiers in Immunology* showed that CRP can be an indicator of chronic inflammatory diseases such as cardiovascular disease, type II diabetes, macular degeneration, and others. Once again tracking blood work, including CRP levels, over time is more useful than relying on a one-time value.

Any level of hs-CRP over 1 mg/L indicates inflammation. It is important to identify and decrease the inflammation that this test indicates is occurring in the body. Lifestyle changes such as the recommendations in this book can help you reduce inflammation naturally.

hs-CRP or high-sensitivity CRP is more sensitive than quantitative CRP and can indicate heart-related inflammation in addition to general inflammation.

Homocysteine

Optimal levels <7.0 umol/L

Homocysteine is an amino acid. Vitamins B6, B9 (folate), and B12 break down this amino acid to create other compounds the body needs to be healthy. Homocysteine is often high if B6, B9, or B12 are too low. It may also be an indicator of a genetic variation called MTHFR or methylene tetrahydrofolate reductase.

If a person has the MTHFR genetic expression the body may have difficulty neutralizing toxins. You may notice that the detergent aisle or perfume department makes you feel ill or cause headaches. The MTHFR genetic indicator can be identified by genetic testing.

Ferritin

Optimal Levels

Male 90–190 ng/mL

Female 80–120 ng/mL

We covered ferritin in the anemia section. When ferritin is low, you have too little stored iron. When ferritin is high we consider it an inflammation marker also known as an acute phase reactant. That is why when the body is in an inflammatory (acute) phase, ferritin levels will react or rise.

IF INFLAMMATION MARKERS ARE HIGH

Inflammation is necessary to help the body heal but if the inflammation becomes chronic it can be the basis of many other disease processes.

FIND THE SOURCE

The most common sources of inflammation are:

- Foods
- Leaky Gut
- Infection
- Toxins
- Stress

INFLAMMATION FROM FOOD

Depending on the individual and his or her ability to digest food adequately, there are many foods that can cause inflammation.

Refined and added sugar is one of the most common foods to cause inflammation. A 2014 study in *JAMA Internal Medicine* found an association between a high-sugar diet and an increased risk of dying from heart disease, which is an inflammatory condition often correlating with a high hs-CRP level. When sugar enters the cells, energy can be produced. If there is an overabundance of sugar it will stay in the bloodstream. In the bloodstream, sugar can cause damage to the lining of the blood vessels. This has the potential to contribute to heart disease. High blood sugar over time causes diabetes and can damage the nerves of the body. According to an August 2019 article in Current Diabetes Report, 50% of adults with diabetes during their lifetime will be affected with neuropathy that can contribute to pain, ulcers, and even lower leg amputation. If that doesn't scare you into curbing your sugar intake, I don't know what will.

If you have an allergy or a sensitivity to a food it can cause inflammation. You may be well aware of a food allergy or sensitivity if you get hives, scratchy throat, upset stomach, or any other body discomfort. You also may not be aware of it since many foods can cause inflammation in the intestinal lining without any overt symptoms. Testing for food sensitivities is covered in Section Ten. Avoid any foods you are sensitive to.

Other foods groups that can be beneficial for the majority of people but may cause inflammation in some individuals:

- Oxalates (wheat, potatoes, spinach)
- Polyphenols (fruit, vegetables, whole grains)
- Gluten (wheat, rye, barley)
- Phytates (beans, seeds, nuts)
- Lectins (legumes, grains, nightshade vegetables)
- Tannins (coffee, tea, wine)
- Glucosinolates (cabbage, kale, cauliflower)
- Saponins (beans, lentils)
- Solanines (potatoes, tomatoes, eggplant)
- Salicylates (broccoli, cauliflower, mushrooms)
- Toxins (advanced glycation end products, trans fats, glycotoxins)

It's always best to work with a health practitioner when removing a food group from your diet. They will know to watch for any significant nutrient deficiencies while you are healing.

INFLAMMATION FROM A LEAKY GUT

Your gut consists of the tube that travels from your mouth to your anus. The lining is what separates the outside world (the inside of the tube) from the inside of your body and blood stream. The cells that line the intestinal wall are like soldiers standing shoulder to shoulder not allowing any foreign particle, virus, bacteria, toxin or overly large or undigested food particle in. Problems arise when the cells pull away from each other and the particles that you would normally poop out gain entry to the body and blood stream. This is called leaky gut or intestinal permeability. Many things can cause the separation of the cells such as vitamin D or other nutrient deficiencies, non steroidal anti-inflammatory drugs, bacteria, viruses, stress, toxins, and organ dysfunction. A leaky gut contributes to nutritional deficiencies, food sensitivities, and more inflammation by triggering autoimmune reactions in the body.

INFLAMMATION FROM INFECTION AND TOXINS

This is where inflammation is often the good guy. Inflammation is the body's immune response to foreign invaders. Sometimes the infection is more difficult to resolve as in the case of Lyme disease, Epstein-Barr virus, or Mono. Toxin exposure can also cause a protective inflammatory reaction that if left unresolved can cause further damage. Removing the infection or toxin is key.

INFLAMMATION FROM STRESS

Stress can be physical like a cut or a bruise, or emotional like worry, grief, or fear. Cortisol, cytokines and other chemicals are released in the body in response to stress and can cause inflammation. Your adrenal glands are affected by stress and can become overworked. It is important to support your adrenal glands with proper nutrition and stress management techniques.

IF FERRITIN LEVELS ARE HIGH

Optimal range for females is 50–150 and for males 75–150.

High ferritin levels may indicate inflammation or other conditions such as too much iron, liver disease, or too much alcohol.

IF HOMOCYSTEINE LEVELS ARE HIGH

Optimal level is < 8 umol/L

Just like sugar, homocysteine levels in the blood can cause damage to the lining of the blood vessels. When this happens the body sends fatty deposits of LDL cholesterol to the injured blood vessel site to help repair it. This process involves inflammation, and the plaques that build up can cause a blockage or they can break off, causing a blockage elsewhere that results in an increased risk of cardiovascular disease.

B6, B12, and folate break down homocysteine, and a high homocysteine level indicates a need for these B vitamins. Foods higher in the amino acid glycine, such as organ meats and bone broth, can also help reduce homocysteine levels.

IF ERYTHROCYTE SEDIMENTATION RATE IS HIGH

Optimal rate is <10 mm/hr

ESR, another inflammation marker, is the time in which your blood cells take to fall to the bottom of a vial in an hour of time. The slower the better. Inflammation causes the red blood cells to be sticky, clump together and fall faster.

FIBRINOGEN

Optimal levels are 175–425 mg/dL

When blood changes from a liquid substance to a more gel-like substance it is called clotting. Blood clots can stop the flow of blood to vital organs and tissues. Fibrinogen levels reflect clotting activity and just like ferritin, it can be a marker of inflammation because it is also an acute phase reactant. Acute phase reactants are proteins indicating inflammation. Fibrinogen has also been shown to be higher in Type 2 diabetes.

VITAMIN D

Optimal levels are 70–90 ng/mL

A 2014 study in the *Journal of Inflammation Research* showed that there is a connection with low vitamin D and inflammatory diseases. Low levels of vitamin D are also associated with insulin resistance and specific muscle weaknesses.

AUTOIMMUNITY

"Autoimmune illness: When you are your own worst enemy."
—Dr. Stacey

Autoimmune reactions are a common source of fatigue and brain fog. This is why I have you look at the thyroid antibody tests, thyroperoxidase (TPO) and thyroglobulin (TgAb) antibodies since thyroid autoimmunity is so common and a common cause of fatigue.

Most autoimmune reactions start in the gut. If there is a leaky gut or intestinal permeability, the toxins, microbes, and undigested food can get into the bloodstream and elicit an immune response. This immune response causes the immune system to not only target the foreign or irritating substance, but to also target the body's own tissues. This immune response causes inflammation. That is why the best protocol for autoimmune conditions is the same as the protocol for inflammation.

Another cause of autoimmunity is stress. 70% of your body's neurotransmitter dopamine, the happy brain chemical, is made in the gut. The transport is up and down the longest nerve in the body, the vagus nerve, which connects the gastrointestinal system to the brain. This is also why you feel "butterflies" in your stomach when you are nervous. A 2009 study in the publication *Autoimmune Reviews* reports that stress causes an immune response that produces inflammatory cytokines that contribute to autoimmunity. Addressing stress using mindful movement, meditation, deep breathing, exercising, prayer, counseling, journaling, and other tools should be implemented for a complete autoimmunity protocol.

DOUSING THE FIRE

There are many aspects to decreasing inflammation. Here are some important steps:

1. Remove the cause (toxins, trauma, sensitivities, viruses, bacteria)
2. Avoid sugar
3. De-stress (mindful movement, journaling, counseling, meditation, deep breathing)
4. Increase nutrients (B vitamins, Vitamin C, Vitamin D, vegetables at every meal, turmeric, ginger, and other herbs)
5. Increase omega-3 oils (wild-caught fish oil, walnuts, flax seed, chia seed, hemp seed)
6. Remove food sensitivities (gluten, dairy, sugar, corn, soy, nuts, eggs, and alcohol are common)

The best foods to decrease inflammation:

- Grass-fed meat and poultry
- Lemons and limes
- Berries
- Green tea
- Avocado
- Ginger
- Garlic
- Turmeric root
- Wild caught SMASH fish (salmon, mackerel, anchovies, sardines, herring)

- Low glycemic or non-starchy vegetables
- Bone broth

The root cause of most diseases is the body trying to protect you with a normal and healthy response that goes on for too long called chronic inflammation. Identify if you have it, search for why it's there and correct the root problem. The subject of inflammation is vast and will be covered another time.

When I was in middle school, my mom went from listening to the current health news of the time to reading *Prevention Magazine*. She switched out sugary desserts after dinner to grapefruit halves. Noodles or rice in my dad's chili were swapped for green beans. And she made us eat a salad before our dinner every evening. She found a healthy balance between her jello masterpieces and luscious chocolate cream pies with fruit and vegetables. I may have complained at the time but I am grateful now. She knew how to incorporate antiinflammatory foods into our diet and help our family take a step in the right "nutrition-rich" direction.

OPTIMAL LAB VALUES FOR INFLAMMATION

hs-CRP	<1.0 mg/L
Fibrinogen	200–400 mg/dL
Sed Rate	Male <50 0–15, >50 0–20mm
	Female <50 0–20, >50 0–30mm
Homocysteine	<7.0 umol/L
25 OH Vitamin D	50–90 ng/mL

CHAPTER HIGHLIGHTS

★ Inflammation is your body's way of protecting you.

★ When inflammation occurs throughout the body over a long period of time, it becomes a risk factor for many disease processes.

★ CRP is a compound released from the liver when inflammation is present.

★ Homocysteine is often high if B6, B9, or B12 are too low. It may also be an indicator of a genetic variation called MTHFR.

★ That is why when the body is in an inflammatory (acute) phase, ferritin levels will react or rise.

★ Refined and added sugar is one of the most common foods to cause inflammation.

★ A leaky gut contributes to nutritional deficiencies, food sensitivities, and inflammation by triggering autoimmune reactions.

★ Steps to decreasing inflammation may include removing the cause, avoiding sugar and food sensitivities, decreasing stress, increasing nutrients, and increasing omega-3 oils.

SECTION SEVEN

PLANNING +
TROUBLESHOOTING =
SUCCESS

"If you don't have a plan and leave your food choices to chance, chances are good that those choices will stink."

—Kristen Bentson

CHAPTER 26

MEAL PLANNING

Don't overthink your meals. It's easy to grab two hard boiled eggs, a handful of carrots and celery and call it a meal. You can also run to your favorite Mexican restaurant for an order of fajitas or a burrito bowl. You can throw bok choy and scallions into some chicken broth, bring it to a boil and whisk in some eggs for a simple and delicious egg drop soup (remember to add a touch of sesame oil).

Many people say they find it difficult to include one to two cups of vegetables in every meal. If you are not a morning vegetable person, add an extra cup of vegetables to lunch and dinner. You can add frozen riced cauliflower and spinach to a smoothie, a smoothie bowl, or breakfast casserole and barely notice it. It can be the base to many dishes. You can use a grilled, lengthwise-sliced zucchini as a base and cover it with taco meat, salsa and guacamole. You can top a large slice of roasted cauliflower with pizza sauce, mozzarella cheese, peppers, and mushrooms. It's not finger food, but it's delicious.

The meal plans I have created for you are low or no cheese and gluten-free due to them being high inflammatory foods for many people. If you know you have a sensitivity, avoid these foods. If you know you don't have a sensitivity, feel free to use dairy as a condiment and, for vegetarians, a protein source. It is still recommended to avoid gluten. Some of the breakfasts do not have vegetables so you can add them to breakfast on the side or you can add an extra cup or two of vegetables to your other meals.

You can also be creative and channel Gordon Ramsey with delicious whole food ingredients.

Have fun with it, discover your inner chef and have on-the-go and simple meals as a back up.

PICK YOUR PREFERENCE

The simplest way to create meals is to start with your list of proteins and your list of vegetables and simply cook them separately or together. Add a healthy oil for dressing, roasting, or sauteing. Add a heavier carb and/or a fruit if that is part of your meal.

Choose organic, grass-fed, or wild-caught.

Protein (choose one serving per meal, 10–20 grams of protein)	Vegetables (choose two servings per meal, ½–1 cup each)	Healthy fat (choose one serving per meal, 1T per serving)	Heavier carb (up to 2 servings a day, ½ cup each)	Fruit (up to 2 servings a day, ½ cup each)
Eggs	Greens	Olive oil	Potato	Berries
Seafood	Broccoli	Ghee	Rice	Apple
Poultry	Cauliflower	Avocado oil	Quinoa	Pear
Beef	Green beans	Olives	Buckwheat	Orange
Legumes	Bell Peppers	Avocado	Beets	Kiwi
etc.	etc.	etc.	etc.	etc.

SMOOTHIES and SMOOTHIE BOWLS

Smoothies are a great way to get a quick protein meal, and a high-speed blender is a great investment for a smooth and not chunky smoothie. A smoothie bowl is typically a blend of the protein, milk, and vegetable poured into a bowl with the nuts, seeds, and fruit added to the top.

Protein	Milk	Healthy Fats	Fruit or vegetable
Hemp hearts	Cow's milk	Nuts	Berries
Pea protein powder	Goat's milk	Seeds	Banana
Whey protein powder	Nut milk	Avocado	Frozen riced cauliflower
Nut or seed butter	Hemp milk	Flax seed	Spinach
Yogurt	Water	Chia seed	Peaches

SOUPS

Soups are a great way to create a meal. It's an easy way to include vegetables, is quick to assemble, makes you feel full longer, and cooked vegetables are typically gentle on the digestive tract.

Chicken, beef, vegetable, and fish broth are all easily found at local supermarkets, or make your own using a crockpot or pressure cooker and whole ingredients. Choose organic, grass-fed, or wild-caught.

30-DAY MEAL PLAN

When creating this 30-day meal plan I wanted to include a variety of foods so you aren't bored of the same meals day in and day out. Saying that, I have found that many people find comfort in repeating meals they love. I personally can eat smoked salmon and cauli-thins (a bread-like substitute made from cauliflower, eggs, and parmesan cheese) every damn day and be perfectly happy.

You will notice that each meal has one serving of protein and two vegetables, and each day has two servings of fruit and two servings of heavier carbs like potato or rice. Feel free to switch them out with other foods of the same category. Although I don't always include the fat or oil in a meal, include a serving from your healthy fat list when you are cooking or sauteing if you aren't using it as a spread or for flavor.

You are welcome to switch out the animal proteins for vegetarian proteins at any time. Take note of what meals make you feel good and sustain you for the next three to four hours. If you feel brain fog or lethargy after a meal try to figure out why. Is it the food, the quantity or something else?

Remember a serving of protein should give you 15 to 20 grams of protein per serving, and a serving of low glycemic vegetables is a half to one cup, whereas the higher glycemic vegetables (corn, potatoes and root vegetables like beets) and fruit are a half cup per serving. Fats and oils are one tablespoon per serving.

I added restaurant meals for Saturday night on the meal plan since that is the night most people eat out if they are going to eat out. You could also make the same meals at home by looking up a low carb recipe.

VARIETY IS THE SPICE OF LIFE

You will see many meals repeated with variations. This is because they provide the nutrients needed in accessible, easy meals. I love great foods with a variety of flavors. If you want to make your meal plans super simple you can add premade sauces with high quality, clean ingredients to your protein and vegetables of choice.

Some sauce companies that get my seal of approval are:

- Primal Kitchen
- Thrive Market
- Fody
- Kevin's
- Eden
- Noble Made
- Core and Rind

You can also make your own or combine ingredients to create great flavor and variety. Here are some:

HUMMUS

Hummus is often a go-to for convenience and creamy goodness. It's made of iron-rich chickpeas and tahini and antioxidant-rich, anti-inflammatory olive oil. While plain ol' hummus is great and delicious, you can create more variety by simply adding a few herbs or spices. Four ounces of hummus is approximately eight grams of protein. Not the 15–20 grams that is recommended per meal so make sure you bump up the protein in other meals.

To 8 oz. of your favorite plain hummus, add and blend:

- Roasted red pepper: 1–2 roasted red peppers
- Sun-dried tomato: ¼ cup sun dried tomatoes, chopped
- Cilantro: ½ cup fresh chopped cilantro
- Roasted garlic: ½ head of roasted garlic
- Dill pickle: ½ cup chopped dill pickles
- Kalamata olive: ¼ cup pitted, kalamata olives
- Lemon: 2 tbsp. lemon zest
- Jalapeño peach: 1 minced jalapeño (minus seeds and ribs, unless you want it hotter) and 2 minced ripe peaches
- Smokey paprika: 1 tbsp. smoked paprika

SMOOTHIES

Protein smoothies can provide the extra protein you need in a day. Don't skimp on your protein! You can use protein powder made from whey, egg white, pea protein, pumpkin seed, hemp, bone broth, and others. Just make sure they don't contain artificial sweeteners like sucralose or inflammatory oils like vegetable oils. Choose a protein powder that has less than ten grams of carbohydrate per serving and at least ten grams of protein. Adding unsweetened cocoa powder or frozen strawberries can decrease the sweetness of a too sweet protein powder. If it isn't sweet enough, add erythritol, allulose, monk fruit, or stevia to taste.

You can include your vegetable serving in a smoothie. Great choices for this are:

- Spinach
- Cauliflower (fresh or frozen)
- Kale
- Carrots
- Summer squash
- Zucchini
- Butternut squash
- Steamed peas (great paired with mint)
- Celery (great paired with apple)
- Cucumber (great paired with pineapple)

Avocado and cooked sweet potato can make a smoothie thick and creamy without adding any dairy or bananas.

To one serving of vanilla protein powder, 8 oz. unsweetened milk or milk substitute, and a dash of sea salt, add and blend:

- Blueberry Bliss: 1 cup fresh spinach + ½ cup frozen blueberries
- Strawberry Supreme: ½ cup frozen cauliflower + ½ cup fresh strawberries
- Spiced Almond: ½ cup frozen yellow summer squash + 1 tbsp. almond butter + ½ tsp. cinnamon
- Mocha Madness: ½ cup frozen cauliflower + 2 tsp. instant decaf coffee + 1 tbsp. cocoa powder
- ChocoAvo: ¼ frozen avocado + 1 tbsp. cocoa powder
- Cherry Chocolate: 1 cup fresh spinach + ½ cup frozen cherries + 1 tbsp. cocoa powder

- Minty Delight: 1 cup fresh spinach + 7 mint leaves + ¼ tsp. vanilla extract
- Carrot Spice: ½ cup frozen shredded carrot + 1 tsp. freshly grated ginger + ½ tsp. cinnamon + ½ tsp. nutmeg + 5 toasted pecans

OMELETTES

Eggs are a perfect food. They often get a bad rap because the yolks contain cholesterol, but cholesterol is needed by the body to make sex hormones (estrogen and testosterone) and stress hormones (cortisol). Eggs contain many nutrients necessary for eye health, blood sugar balance, and muscle maintenance. Three whole eggs supplies approximately 18 grams of protein. You can choose egg whites only, if you prefer. Five to six egg whites or a three-quarter cup gives you approximately 20 grams of protein. Another option is to have two eggs with one meal and increase your protein in another meal that day. The variety of egg dishes is endless. Many omelettes contain cheese. You are welcome to include an ounce of cheese as a serving of fat for these high protein dishes as long as you don't have a sensitivity to dairy.

Here are a few non-dairy favorites.

To 3 eggs or ¾ cup of egg whites and sea salt to taste cooked in a skillet, add:

- Florentine: 1 cup sauteed spinach + 2 tbsp. hollandaise sauce

- Mexican: ½ cup sauteed bell pepper + ½ cup sauteed onion + 3 tbsp. salsa
- Italian: 1 tbsp. tomato sauce + 1 oz. cooked ground sausage + ¼ tsp. oregano
- Spring: ½ cup sauteed mushrooms + ½ cup spring peas + ¼ tsp. chopped fresh dill
- Omega: 2 oz. smoked salmon + thinly sliced red pepper + ¼ tsp. chopped fresh dill
- Extra Omega: 2 oz. sardine + 1 cup sauteed spinach + hot sauce
- Southwestern: ½ cup sauteed onion + ½ cup sauteed chopped tomato + ¼ avocado + ¼ tsp. chili powder
- Asian: ½ cup sauteed bok choy + ½ cup sauteed shiitake mushrooms + green onion + ¼ tsp. sesame oil

SHAKSHUKA

Shakshuka, meaning mixture, is a dish that originated in North Africa but gained popularity in the Middle East and is basically eggs poached in a sea of vegetables. Most known for the tomato-based version, it can be any combination of any sauteed vegetables.

Saute the vegetables in a pan over medium heat until soft, stirring occasionally. While simmering, create a few divots in the sauce. Crack an egg into each divot. Reduce the heat to low and cover for 6 to 10 minutes or until the eggs are done to your satisfaction. Salt and pepper to taste.

Don't feel limited to only using eggs as the protein in this dish. You can use wild-caught fish, tofu, lentils, or chickpeas as well as any other protein that sounds good to you.

Here are a few variations:

- Traditional: tomatoes, peppers, garlic, and onions + paprika, cumin, and chili powder
- Spinach pie: spinach, green onion, parsley, feta and garlic
- Root: carrots, parsnip, sweet potato, butternut squash + nutmeg and cinnamon
- Curry: tomatoes, onion, ginger, garlic, and eggplant + curry powder
- Arti-olive: tomatoes, onion, artichoke, olives + oregano and garlic powder
- Go Green: spinach, onion, garlic, zucchini, and peas + basil, rosemary, and thyme
- Southwest: tomatoes, onion, peppers, olives, and garlic + cumin and chili powder
- Asian: bokchoy, onion, spinach, mushroom + soy sauce and sesame oil

HOT HEMP CEREAL

As comforting as oatmeal but loaded with heart-healthy omega oils, hemp hearts, chia, and flax seeds create a powerful combination in this hot cereal. Combine ¼ cup hemp hearts, ¼ cup chia seeds, and 1 tablespoon flax seed with 1 cup unsweetened milk of choice in a saucepan over medium high heat for approximately 5 minutes stirring frequently. Add a natural sweetener like monk fruit, erythritol or allulose to taste. Spice it up with cinnamon, nutmeg, ginger, cardamom, cocoa powder, lemon zest, or other natural flavor.

WRAPS

Who doesn't love a good sandwich? It's easy to put together and a popular lunch option. I want to help you forgo the bread and grains that typically make up a sandwich with vegetable and protein-focused options.

It can be as simple as a leaf of lettuce to a complex recipe with coconut and almond flour. I have seen wraps made from carrot, coconut, and jicama. There are many grain-free, lower-carb recipes online that would work for a wrap. Check them out.

Anything you would use to construct a sandwich can be used with these wrap ideas. I gave you some ideas in the meal plan.

My favorite options are:
- Lettuce wraps: Romaine is my go-to, but some prefer Boston Bib lettuce or cabbage leaves.
- Cauliflower thins: Made from eggs, cauliflower, and parmesan cheese and yeast, I love to pair these with smoked salmon and everything-but-the-bagel-seasonings from Trader Joe's.
- Crepini: Made with cauliflower, eggs, and olive oil, these are my new favorite wraps, lasagna noodles, soup noodles, and so much more. Although they can tear easily, I am loving these wraps!

- Maria Emmerich's tortilla recipe: Super easy recipe made from egg whites. This is a great way to get more protein. I've included the recipe below.

Maria Emmerich's Tortilla Recipe (www.mariamindbodyhealth.com):

- ➤ 2 egg whites
- ➤ Pinch of cream of tartar
- ➤ ⅛ tsp. sea salt (Maria prefers Redmond's Real Salt)
- ➤ 1 tsp. powdered Allulose (a sugar free natural sweetener)
- ➤ 1 tbsp. unflavored egg white powder

Preheat the oven to 325 degrees F. Line baking sheets with parchment paper. Spray the parchment with avocado oil spray.

Place the egg whites, cream of tartar, salt and allulose in a food processor, blender, or a bowl using a hand mixer.

Mix on high until the whites double in size and there are soft peaks. Add the egg white powder and blend until just combined.

Use a spatula to spread the mix out on the prepared baking sheets as thin as you can, about ⅛ inch thick.

Place into the oven to bake for 6–8 minutes or until cooked though.

Remove from the oven and let it cool completely. Once cool, gently peel the parchment paper off.

Fill with anything.

Variations:

- Beef sauteed with ginger, garlic, coconut aminos, a tea-spoon of peanut butter, and sesame oil with shredded carrots and bok choy
- Falafel, tomatoes, cucumbers, and yogurt with dill and lemon juice
- Tuna salad with diced carrots, cucumber, onion, tomato, and olive oil or mayonnaise.
- Egg salad with diced onions, celery, and olive oil or may-onnaise
- Reuben: corned beef, sauerkraut, and homemade Rus-sian dressing
- Turkey, tomato, and avocado
- Meatballs and marinara sauce with roasted peppers and onions
- Grilled chili-spiced cod, salsa, and cabbage

CASSEROLES

My Aunt Marge used to make the best tuna rice casserole. I would even ask for it for my birthday. Nothing says comfort like a fresh-out-of-the-oven casserole. Our healthy versions will have a variety of protein, vegetables, and spices. The sauce makes it creamy without dairy. If you mix an egg into the base it will hold the ingredients together like a souffle. The sauce is mixed into the spiced protein and vegetable mix and baked in the oven.

Preheat your oven to 350 degrees F.

Layer your cooked protein and fresh vegetables in a greased casserole dish. Sprinkle the spices on top. Cover and bake for 30 minutes. Alternatively you can saute vegetables in a pan on the stove and add to a casserole dish.

While the protein and vegetables are baking, heat 2 tablespoons of avocado oil in a saucepan over medium heat.

Add in 2 tablespoons coconut flour and 2 tablespoons almond flour. Cook and stir until all the flour turns dark brown and absorbs all the oil. This will take about 1 minute.

Pour in 1 cup of unsweetened coconut milk or almond milk, stirring constantly. Once it boils, reduce heat to low. Cook for 10 minutes or until the sauce thickens, stirring often enough that it doesn't burn. Season to taste. Take the saucepan off the stove and let cool briefly. Whisk in one egg.

Remove the casserole from the oven, uncover, and gently mix in the sauce. Return it to the oven uncovered and bake for another 45 minutes. Allow 10 minutes to cool before serving. Season to taste.

Variations:

- Chili-spiced Turkey: 1 lb cooked ground turkey + 1 cup sliced onion + 1 cup sliced bell pepper + 1 cup sliced summer squash + 1 ½ cup tomato sauce + 3 cloves minced garlic + ½ tsp. cumin + 1 tsp. chili powder + 1 tsp. sea salt

- Chicken and Root Vegetables: 1 lb cooked chicken breast + 1 cup sliced onion + 1 cup thinly sliced sweet potato + 1 cup diced parsnip + 1 cup diced beets + 1 tsp. ground thyme + 1 tsp. sea salt
- Asian Beef: Beef + 1 garlic clove + 1 tsp. ginger + 1 tbsp. peanut butter + 2 tsp. sesame oil + 1 tsp. hot sauce
- Dijon Steak: 1 lb seasoned steak, cooked and sliced + 2 cups cauliflower florets + 1 cup sliced bell pepper + 1 cup sliced onion + 4 cloves minced garlic + 1 tbsp. dijon mustard mixed with 1 tbsp. coconut aminos + 1 tsp. oregano
- Bacon Chicken: 1 lb diced roasted chicken breast + ½ lb cooked bacon, crumbled + 12 oz. riced cauliflower + 1 cup sliced onion + 2 cups broccoli florets + 2 tbsp. nutritional yeast + 1 tsp. sea salt + ½ tsp. black pepper
- Tuna "Rice": 2 cans skipjack tuna + 1 cup diced onion + 1 cup diced green pepper + 1 cup sliced mushrooms + 12 oz. riced cauliflower + 1 tsp. thyme + 1 tsp. sea salt + 1 tsp. black pepper
- Shepherd's Pie: 1 lb ground lamb + 1 cup green peas + 1 cup diced green beans. Top with 12 oz. mashed potatoes or mashed cauliflower

SOUP

I am a lazy soup maker. I throw everything into a pot with broth and pressure cook it for ten minutes, but you can also put it in a pot and let it sit on the stove for an hour. Voila, done! My favorite shortcut is pre-cut carrots, celery, and onion called mirepoix.

You can find it at most grocery stores or happily chop them yourself. The following are some of my favorite combinations.

Saute 1 large, chopped onion, 2–3 stalks chopped celery, 3 chopped carrots, and 2 cloves minced garlic in butter or olive oil until fragrant, then add 8 cups of broth and these ingredients:

- Italian Wedding: 12 oz. (organic, grass-fed) chicken, turkey, beef, or plant-based meatballs, 1 tbsp. oregano, ¼ cup parmesan, ¼ cup chopped parsley, 4 cups chopped fresh spinach
- Lemon Turkey: 2 cups cooked and diced organic turkey, 1 chopped red pepper, 1 cup chopped fresh spinach, ½ cup chopped parsley, ½ cup chopped cilantro, juice of one lemon, zest of one lemon
- Mushroom and Vegetable: 8 oz. fresh mushrooms (shiitake, button, cremini, portabella, or combination), 1 cup chopped zucchini, 1 chopped orange pepper, 1 cup cherry tomatoes
- Green Pepper Vegetable: 1 green pepper chopped, 1 summer squash diced, 1 cup tomatoes chopped, ¼ cup chopped cilantro and ¼ cup chopped parsley
- West African Peanut: 2 medium sweet potatoes, diced, 1 cup smooth peanut butter, 1 cup diced tomatoes, 14.5 oz. tomato sauce, 1 tsp. cumin, ½ tsp. ginger
- Egg Drop: Omit mirepoix. 3 green onion chopped, 4 scrambled eggs poured into the boiling soup in a steady thin stream while whisking. 1 tbsp. soy sauce, 1 tbsp. sesame oil

- Sesame Bok Choy: Omit mirepoix. ½ inch of ginger, grated, 1 head of bok choy, chopped, 1 tbsp. sesame oil
- Chicken Lemon "Rice": Omit mirepoix. 3 cups cooked, diced chicken, 2 cups riced cauliflower, scramble 4 eggs with juice of 4 lemons and slowly add to simmering broth, one tbsp. at a time, whisking constantly for a smooth consistency

You can use an immersion blender to make a "creamier" soup or add coconut milk or cream for a creamed soup.

Always season to taste.

BUDDHA BOWLS

When you throw protein, veggies, healthy fats, and a touch of carbs in a bowl, it looks like Buddha's big belly to me (and it sure fills up my belly), hence "Buddha Bowls." For these bowls I love to include a fermented vegetable for some much needed probiotics. Kimchi, sauerkraut, or other fermented vegetables are great choices. Although pickles can be fermented, don't confuse "pickled" with "fermented." Both preserve food but pickling uses an acidic brine whereas fermentation uses beneficial bacteria or yeast. Beneficial bacteria is good for gut health and brain health so include fermented foods whenever possible.

Here are some wonderful Buddha Bowl combinations:

- Chinese: ¼ lb ground organic / grass-fed beef + fermented kimchi + whisk together: 1 tbsp. peanut butter, 1 tbsp. coconut aminos, 1 clove garlic, minced, 1 tsp.

grated ginger, 1 tsp. sesame oil, 1 tsp. rice vinegar + ½ cup quinoa
- Middle Eastern: Falafel + hummus + tahini + fermented pickles and radishes
- Mediterranean: Lentils + fermented sauerkraut + lemon, tahini, olive oil dressing + ½ diced sweet potato
- Japanese: Wild-caught Ahi tuna + fermented vegetable mix + crumbled seaweed + rice vinegar + ½ cup rice

SALADS

Never hesitate to grab a bagged salad from the grocery store and call it a day. It never ceases to amaze me how many salad options are now available. Be adventurous and try something new. If you are a DIY kind of person, here are some tried-and-true salad variations:

- Cobb: turkey + egg + mixed greens + cherry tomatoes + red wine vinegar
- Greek: grilled chicken + mixed greens + red onions + cucumbers + olives + fermented radishes + oregano/red wine vinegar/olive oil
- Italian: chickpeas + mixed greens + parsley + pepperoncini + olives + artichokes + cucumber + tomato + red wine vinegar/ garlic/ olive oil
- Middle Eastern: lentils + mixed greens + grilled eggplant + grilled peppers + grilled onions + tahini/lemon/olive oil
- Nicoise: tuna + green beans + hard boiled egg + tomatoes + olives + dijon mustard/olive oil/ white wine vinegar/ shallots

- Poke: ahi tuna + mixed greens + avocado + pickled ginger + crumbled dried seaweed + toasted sesame seeds
- Taco: ground organic / grass-fed beef + mixed greens + salsa + sour cream
- Ranch: steak + mixed greens + tomato + avocado + red onion + blue cheese + ranch dressing

"ON THE GO"

CONVENIENT FOODS

Whether you are on a field trip, going cross country or just traveling to and from work, make sure you have healthy convenience foods in your car or backpack to avoid skipping meals. (choose organic, grass-fed, or wild-caught animal proteins)

- Jerky, beef, or turkey sticks (nitrate-free, grass fed)
- Kale chips
- Seaweed snack packs
- Roasted crunchy peas
- Hard boiled eggs
- Cut up veggies
- Apples
- Oranges
- Guacamole cups
- Salsa cups
- Olive packs
- Pickle packs
- Roasted crunchy lentils

- Unsweetened applesauce cups
- Cheese sticks
- Pork rinds
- Unsweetened yogurt cups
- Nuts (walnuts, pistachio, almonds, etc.)
- Seeds (pumpkin, sunflower, hemp, etc.)
- Protein bars
- Protein shakes
- Tuna (choose wild-caught skipjack) packs

RESTAURANTS

Choose restaurants with a variety of fresh, and not canned, vegetables. Farm-to-table restaurants typically have the freshest whole food options because they get their food straight from the farm. Most restaurants have egg dishes like omelets which are always a good choice. Organic eggs would be preferable, so if you can find a restaurant that serves organic, choose that one.

Steak House

Steak with fresh vegetable side dishes and a salad is a good choice. Typically they also have chicken and fish options as well.

Japanese

Rice is a large part of Japanese dishes. Choose more protein and vegetable heavy dishes. Some sushi restaurants now offer sushi rolls without rice.

Middle Eastern

Kebabs are a great choice. So is hummus with vegetables to dip.

Korean

Bibimbap is typically a protein, vegetable, and rice dish served in a piping hot stone bowl with an egg on top. It's a great choice with the rice or with extra vegetables and no rice.

Mexican

Fajitas are a great choice at Mexican restaurants. Plenty of protein and vegetables make this dish an easy win.

Indian

Tandoori and tikka dishes with the sauces on the side provide excellent protein. Punjabi eggplant is a great vegetable option.

FAST FOOD

Fast food joints should be avoided at all costs due to the dangerous trans fats, high sodium, fillers, and additives in menu items. When it's your only option you want to make it work and make the best choices. Avoid the refined-carbohydrate buns, the high-inflammatory oil-soaked fries and the sweet stuff.

Consider that the ingredient list for grilled chicken in a well-loved and popular fast food restaurant is not just chicken.

The ingredient list reads like a novel:

Chicken (boneless, skinless chicken breast, water, apple cider vinegar, soybean oil, modified corn starch, salt, yeast extract, sugar, chicken breast meat, chicken broth, dehydrated onion, dehydrated garlic, sea salt, cane molasses, spices, chicken fat, natural flavor [including smoke], lemon peel, red bell pepper, paprika, lemon juice concentrate, parsley and vinegar solids, xanthan gum, and calcium disodium EDTA [to protect quality])

If you are not going to avoid fast food restaurants no matter what I say, choose:

- Bunless burgers
- Bunless grilled chicken
- Low-carb burrito bowls
- Egg-based meals
- Low-carb salads
- Lettuce wraps
- Unsweetened drinks
- Fresh vegetables whenever available

While fast food should be avoided, there are a few joints I've put on the acceptable list.

Chipotle

Chipotle has great choices and is at the top of my fast food list. I love that it recently added cilantro lime cauliflower rice in some locations. What a great way to satisfy your carb-ish cravings. I celebrate when businesses listen to their customers' requests for healthier choices.

A simple meal of protein and grilled veggies is often enough, but you can add a small serving of beans, rice, or guacamole to create two meals or one really hearty meal.

Skip the chips due to their inflammatory oils and the flour tortillas made from refined flour.

Panera

Panera has great salads and you can create your own lettuce wrap sandwich with turkey, chicken, or ham, bacon and avocado.

Include a slice of whole grain bread if you are including it in your two servings for the day.

Skip the sweets.

Wendy's

Wendy's chili is a good choice. Add a salad to complete the meal.

If it's not listed here, it is not recommended.

Don't make fast food a frequent event, only an exception when you can't find another way.

Action Task: Restaurant Rescue Resource

1. Make a list of restaurants and best choices from those restaurants.
2. Keep it in your phone notes.
3. Review them before ordering. When you are hungry you are less likely to make good decisions.
4. Make a plan for what you will order, and stick to it.

SUN

1: Traditional shakshuka + blackberries
2: Italian wedding soup
3: Beef jerky + veg + orange
4: Chili-seasoned shrimp+ peppers/onions + rice

MON

1: Florentine omelette + blueberries
2: Asian beef lettuce wraps + peach
3: Roasted red pepper hummus + veg + pickles
4: Grilled lamb + green beans/tomatoes + potato

TUES

1: Strawberry supreme smoothie
2: Cobb salad
3: Nut butter + veg + apple
4: Italian spiced squash and lentils

WED

1: Spinach pie shakshuka + blackberries
2: Lemon turkey soup
3: Falafel + veg + kiwi
4: Dijon steak casserole

THURS

1: Cinnamon hot hemp cereal + raspberries
2: Middle East Buddha Bowl
3: Nuts + veg + melon
4: Chicken kebab + peppers/onion + sw. potato

FRI

1: Mexican omelet + blueberries
2: Falafel wrap + pear
3: Sun-dried tomato hummus + veg + pickle
4: Chili-spiced turkey casserole

SAT

1: Blueberry bliss smoothie
2: Greek salad
3: Nut butter + veg + grapes
4: Steakhouse filet mignon + green beans +salad

SUN

1: Root shakshuka + blackberries
2: Mushroom and vegetable soup
3: Falafel + veg + kiwi
4: Mexican fajitas

MON

1: Italian omelette + blueberries
2: Tuna salad wrap + pear
3: Cilantro hummus + veg + pickles
4: Roasted turkey + Br. sproats/carrots + rice

TUES

1: Spiced almond smoothie
2: Italian salad
3: Nut butter + veg + grapes
4: Bun-less chicken burgers +cauli/broccoli

WED

1: Curry shakshuka + blackberries
2: Green pepper vegetable soup
3: Turkey jerky + veg + orange
4: Stuffed peppers

THURS

1: Ginger hot hemp cereal + raspberries
2: Mediterranean Buddha bowl
3: Nuts + veg + plum
4: Turkey meatloaf + brocolli/kale + mash. pot.

FRI

1: Spring omelette + blueberries
2: Egg salad wrap + peach
3: Roasted garlic hummus + veg + pickles
4: Chicken and root vegetable casserole

SAT

1: Mocha madness smoothie
2: Middle Eastern salad
3: Nut butter + veg + apple
4: Japanese sashimi + seaweed + edamame

Week Two

The Supercharged Method

SUN

1: Arti-olive shakshuka + blackberries
2: West African peanut soup
3: Salmon jerky + veg + orange
4: Mexican shrimp + onions/peppers + rice

MON

1: Omega omelette + blueberries
2: Reuben wrap + peach
3: Dill pickle hummus + veg + pickles
4: Lamb stew + celery/onion/carrots/potato

TUES

1: ChocoAvo smoothie
2: Nicoise salad
3: Nut butter + veg + apple
4: Shepard pie casserole

WED

1: Go green shakshuka + blackberries
2: Egg drop soup
3: Falafel + veg + kiwi
4: Mexican beans/rice + onions/tomatoes

THURS

1: Cocoa hot hemp cereal + raspberries
2: Japanese Buddha Bowl
3: Nuts + veg + melon
4: Turkey spaghetti +lentil noodles

FRI

1: Extra omega omelette + blueberries
2: Turkey, tomato & avocado wrap + pear
3: Kalamata olive hummus + veg + pickles
4: Bacon chicken casserole

SAT

1: Cherry chocolate smoothie
2: Poke salad
3: Nut butter + veg + grapes
4: Greek chicken kebabs + grilled veg. + salad

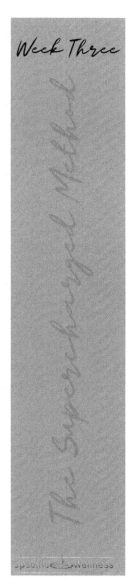

Week Three

The Supercharged Method

Specific Wellness

Week Four

SUN
1: Southwest shakshuka + blackberries
2: Sesame bok choy soup
3: Falafel + veg + kiwi
4: Vegetable loaded beef and bean chili

MON
1: Southwestern omelette + blueberries
2: Meatball wrap with peppers/onions + pear
3: Lemon hummus + veg + pickles
4: Indian Tandoori chicken + grilled veg.

TUES
1: Mint-y delight smoothie
2: Taco salad
3: Nut butter + veg + grapes
4: Scallops + asparagus + grilled red peppers

WED
1: Asian shakshuka + blackberries
2: Chicken lemon "rice" soup
3: Bison jerky + veg + orange
4: Lemon picatta sole + asparagus/kale + rice

THURS
1: Lemony hot hemp cereal + raspberries
2: Chinese Buddha bowl
3: Nuts + veg + plum
4: Rotisserie chicken + cabbage/celery + quinoa

FRI
1: Asian omelette + blueberries
2: Grilled cod wrap + peach
3: Jalapeno peach hummus + veg + pickles
4: Tuna "rice" casserole

SAT
1: Carrot spice smoothie
2: Ranch salad
3: nut butter + veg + apple
4: Korean bibimpap + extra vegetables

The Supercharged Method

CHAPTER HIGHLIGHTS

★ Don't overthink your meals. Keep it simple.

★ Add frozen vegetables to smoothies.

★ Make a list of restaurants and best choices from those restaurants.

★ Choose whole foods whenever possible.

CHAPTER 27

PLAN YOUR MINDSET

I don't know who said it, but the quote, "You have been assigned this mountain to show others it can be moved," resonates with me. Whatever obstacle you are facing, whatever goal you want to achieve, it all starts with you telling yourself it is possible. "Possible" doesn't mean it will happen, but it starts to align the stars in your mind to move towards the actions it will take to get there. Go move those mountains and show others it can be done.

WHY MINDSET IS IMPORTANT

Brenda's Story

When Brenda came in, she had a grocery bag of over 20 supplement bottles that she rarely used. As we went through them, one by one, we discovered that she really didn't know why she was taking most of them. How many times are you given a supplement or medication and you don't know why you are taking it? If you take the time to learn your "why" you may notice you will have a better outcome no matter what it pertains to. Over the next few months I was able to narrow down the supplements she needed most and educate her as to why they were important for her personally. The electrolytes made her leg cramps disappear. The magnesium relieved her headaches. The L-Glutamine resolved her stomach aches. Once she made the connection of what supplements affected her particular conditions she was more apt to take them and actually feel better.

Carol Dweck, the author of *Mindset: The Psychology of Success*, says, "Effort is one of those things that gives meaning to life. Effort means that you care about something, that something is important to you and you are willing to work for it."

This course is easy, but it takes effort. You will only give that effort if you care about what you want to achieve. What is that? You may say it's to have energy. You may say it's to be able to focus. You may say it's to be able to think clearly. It's not any of that. What you really want is along the lines of not having to miss out because you need a nap, or not losing your job because it takes so long to finish a project, or not being terrified that you will injure yourself or someone else when you drive because your brain is full of fluff.

MINDSET MAVENS

I want to introduce you to some coaches and authors that have helped me with my mindset.

I don't know if there is anyone I admire more than the Southern-drawling, swear-like-a-sailor, diet-truth-preaching dynamo Corinne Crabtree. She teaches how to live the life you love while getting your head on straight around food. She lost over 100 pounds, kept it off, and now teaches the masses how to do the same. She teaches you to eat when you are hungry and stop when you have had enough. That seems logical but the real gold is in her guidance around "shitty thoughts." When you can identify the thoughts around why you eat when you are not hungry and why you do not stop at enough, you will have the insight to change your behavior. Not only that but she is generous with a multitude of free podcasts and a free course. You can find her at www.nobsfreecourse.com

If you want to adopt good habits but don't know where to start James Clear has the answer. His book *Atomic Habits* will not only get you to a place to create the habits you want, he also will give you tools to help sustain those habits. James Clear knows not everyone resonates with just one way of doing anything so he gives a multitude of suggestions to create the habits you want. I can thank JC for my nighttime routine that makes my morning plans a no-brainer.

Want a dose of humor while you learn how to meet your goals? Author Jon Acuff is a funny guy. He also wrote a book on the soundtracks we play in our mind that keep us stuck. Literally, it's called *Soundtracks*, and he shows us how to make the thoughts in our head work for us and not against us. He also has a podcast that is motivating and inspirational.

Do you need a kick in the rear? Brooke Castillo, of The Life Coach School, will tell it like it is. If you have goals she will get you there. Her insight that the good stuff in your life is on the other side of being uncomfortable might be familiar but the way she teaches that and other distinctions is innovative and brilliant. Her concept of 50/50 is something that I wish I had learned when I was a kid. 50% of the time you experience good feelings from your life experiences and 50% of the time you will have bad feelings. She teaches that it's normal because life is like that, good and bad experiences. In fact, the good experiences wouldn't feel so good if they didn't have the bad experiences to contrast against. Embracing this idea by allowing ourselves to be uncomfortable while we work through our feelings, instead of resisting and developing bad habits that cause us to numb out, is a game changer.

GET YOUR DUCKS IN A ROW

Some will find that it takes them weeks to just get organized. Go through your cupboards and get rid of any processed, artificial, and high sugar foods. Just do it!! It took me months but my routine looks something like this…

Before bed I will:

- Fill the hot water kettle for green tea in the morning and fill my tumbler or jar with water and electrolytes.
- Make a loaded salad, stir fry, or a shake for meals the next day.
- Set out my work out clothes so I practically trip over them as soon as I enter the hallway.
- Know what workout I will be doing the next morning so I don't have to think about it or scroll through workouts in the morning using brain power I don't yet have.
- Have my daily planner available to prepare for my day and journal.

Planning what I will eat the next day usually includes:

- A quart of water in the morning with lime and erythritol or a packet of electrolytes.
- Green tea.
- A shake or a salad that I eat when my stomach starts growling around noon. The salad consists of mixed greens, ¼ avocado, walnuts, healthy dressing and wild-caught salmon, tuna or organic chicken. The shake is made with protein powder, frozen blueberries, spinach and frozen cauliflower (honestly, you can't even taste it).
- Eggs or another protein and broccoli with butter and sea salt, which I eat around 3 p.m.
- Salmon and roasted vegetables, another shake, or a cup of unsweetened yogurt with berries, brazil nuts, and hemp seed that I eat around 6 p.m. I also eat cut up peppers, tomatoes, carrots, cucumbers, and/or celery at this time.
- I always make a note of what I think I might eat off plan, and I don't make myself feel bad for eating it as long as it doesn't make my energy crash or give me brain fog or gut issues.
- This is subject to change as I'm always trying new meals that have my body functioning at its best.

Is it a dosage issue?

You may notice that your lack of energy may be a dosage issue. One to three chips, you may still be feeling fine. Seven to ten chips make you tired, bloated and frustrated. Note that and go back to baseline before you try it again. Maybe this time try it as part of a meal instead of in the closet at midnight feeding the falling crumbs to the dog. That is me. I'm raising my hand here. My family knows that chips are something that I tend to binge on if I know where they are. We all have our kryptonite and I'm working on mine.

If you are someone who thinks they need to feel full (a thought we should work on) increase your protein and vegetables. Don't eat extra carbs that can spike your blood sugar and make you crash into a post-carb coma. You may be someone who doesn't eat much. In this case, eat one serving of protein and two half-cup servings of veggies at every meal with two to four tablespoons of healthy fat throughout the day and forgo the other options.

If you like to plan:

There are plenty of suggestions in The Supercharged Method to help you plan. If you like to do things on impulse, just know where to find your healthiest choices and avoid places and situations that are going to derail your efforts.

If you know what works for your body, then do what works. If you don't know what to do, start by doing The Supercharged Method.

Anticipate obstacles:

- Write out what could go wrong.
- What situations will cause you to fail?
- What people tend to encourage you to indulge?

- What emotions make your efforts go sideways?
- What scheduling constraints will get in your way? Can you avoid them by preparing food in advance?

HEALTHY HABITS

What habits have served you and which have gotten in your way?

What do you need to reclaim your energy, clarity, and focus? You may say you need to give up the things you love, do the things you hate, and be miserable just trying to get there.

Wrong, wrong, wrong. Let me explain something to you. I've been working with people resolving fatigue and brain fog for over 25 years.

I help people just like you to embrace fun and make healthy, simple changes to supercharge your health. It may be uncomfortable but it doesn't have to be miserable.

If you are in the space of confusion, frustration, and being overwhelmed then let me walk you through the mindset that will make The Supercharged Method feel like a worthwhile challenge.

1. Be open to trying something new. I know it's scary to try something new but what you have been doing up until now hasn't worked. Isn't it time to explore new territory?
2. Be teachable. There are times in our lives where we are open to suggestions and there are times we are not. Where are you? Do you feel you have learned all you can? Do you feel you have explored every aspect of your fatigue and have come to the conclusion that nothing

will work? What if you took off your "knowing" hat and allowed the possibility that The Supercharged Method could, just maybe, work for you?

3. Be curious. Once you take off that "knowing" hat, try putting on your "curiosity" hat. It is an astounding world out there when you choose to be curious. Ask questions. Dig deep. Go down that rabbit hole of information. It's amazing what you might discover about where your fatigue is coming from and what it takes to resolve it. We get bored so easily. Don't let that happen to you during *The Supercharged Method*. If your eyes start glazing over in one section, skip it and go to the next. You might find yourself going back to it once you have delved deeper in other areas.

4. Be brave. There will be times when you will feel scared to change old habits or remove foods you have been dependent on for so long. I promise you, you are brave enough to move past the tools you have used that no longer serve you.

5. Be aware. What are your habits? What changes your mood? What have you tried that worked and what failed? Once you know that, then you can start doing the thought work it takes to meet your goals.

6. Who are you affected by? I developed my habit of eating late at night with my dad and the hot dogs and freezer desserts. Your spouse/partner supports you one minute and sabotages your efforts the next. Your kids bringing in chips and pizza that is just too tempting to pass up from a serious case of fomo. Your family may have snacks

and food that are tempting to you. Learn to eat when you are hungry and stop when you have had enough or, if it contributes to your illness, leave it alone.

7. Fall in love with the process. Shift your attitude from "damn another salad" to "What can I put in this salad that is new and exciting for me? Or comforting?" Some-days I shove 3 cups of mixed greens in a bowl and call it a meal. Other days I will top it with roasted red peppers, marinated artichokes, olives, capers, pickled beets, hard boiled eggs, and avocado. In other words I am either loving getting the job done or loving creating a culinary adventure. Think to yourself, "How can I make today easy and fun on my health quest?"

If you were to stand in your desired future of energy, clarity, and focus:

What would you have to have overcome and how did you over-come it?

_____

_____

What habits and behaviors would you have adopted?

_____

_____

What are you able to accomplish with all this energy, clarity, and focus?

_____

_____

Why was it important to you to overcome your fatigue and brain fog?

_____

_____

CHAPTER HIGHLIGHTS

★ When you can identify the thoughts around why you eat when you are not hungry and why you do not stop at enough, you will have the insight to change your behavior

★ Allow yourself to be uncomfortable while working through feelings instead of resisting and developing bad habits that cause you to numb out.

★ Plan ahead.

★ Work on who you want to be and how you want to feel.

CHAPTER 28

PLAN YOUR MOVEMENT

"Moving your body isn't what you have to do to be healthy,
it's what you get to do to celebrate the health you have."

—Dr. Stacey

Moving your body is important to gain, restore, and maintain energy. There must be a balance of movement that is gentle and calming and challenges your muscles and joints. The varieties of activities all have their place at different times, for different people and situations with different results. If stress rules your life and work or home or life-situations continually make your heart beat faster and your blood pressure rise, the best movement for you would be restorative. If you are sitting all day with minimal stress, basically "chilling" all the time, the best movement for you would challenge your muscles and joints.

RESTORATIVE MOVEMENT

Your body has receptors to constantly monitor your environment, internally (thoughts and body functions) and externally (real and perceived threats). When your brain gets a warning signal, your primitive response is to run or "fight." The fight or flight response is part of your nervous system called the sympathetic nervous system and is called upon when your body perceives danger. In modern times such as these, "danger" ranges from anticipating a physical attack to panic over a deadline and anything in between. When this happens your body will redirect blood from your gastrointestinal tract to your heart, lungs, and muscles. You will notice you are breathing quicker, your heart is beating faster, your pupils dilate (get bigger) to allow more visual input, and your muscles are stronger and quicker. The chemical that initiates all of this is adrenaline. Adrenaline is produced in the adrenal glands which are triangular shaped organs that sit on top of your kidneys. When needed, this system works wonderfully. When it is used over and over again from day-to-day stress it can cause wear and tear of the adrenal glands which can cause them to over or under function, both of which can cause fatigue. Gentle movement and avoiding rigorous movement are one of the many keys in restoring proper adrenal function.

The following are practices that combine body postures, movement, breathing, and meditation for restoration.

- Yoga
- Tai Chi
- Walking
- Qi Gong

CHALLENGING MOVEMENT

If you don't challenge your muscles they become weak. Sitting day in and day out without exercise can cause a breakdown of muscle fibers or atrophy which results in weakness. Muscle weakness can contribute to postural changes, impaired breathing, body aches and pain, and can even set you up for a heart attack.

Your heart is a muscle and making sure that muscle can beat hard and fast when you are under stress and return to a normal rhythm at rest is important to prevent cardiovascular disease. Healthy blood vessels have some elasticity to them and by pumping your blood through at a greater rate, such as when you exercise with more intensity, helps to keep them more flexible.

Resistance training, either with body weight, free weights, machines or resistance bands, and high intensity interval training (HIIT) are recommended.

CHAPTER HIGHLIGHTS

★ Moving your body is important to gain, restore, and maintain energy.

★ Gentle movement and avoiding rigorous movement are one of the many keys in restoring proper adrenal function.

★ If you don't challenge your muscles they become weak.

★ Exercising with more intensity helps to keep blood vessels flexible.

CHAPTER 29

TROUBLESHOOTING FOOD SENSITIVITIES

"It's not you, it's your food"

—Dr. Stacey

TIM'S STORY

Tim has had gut issues for years, but they come and go. He will remove dairy, or some other food, for a while and he feels better. This time he came to me to tell me that his gut was acting up again. He was confused because he said he couldn't narrow it down this time. We went through what he was eating and when he was getting symptoms. He was fine when he ate Mexican and Thai but had symptoms when he ate his vegetable and noodle dish. I asked him what Mexican dishes he favored. He told me tacos. I asked him soft-shell or hard. He told me hard-shell, which are typically corn and not wheat. I asked him what dishes he ate when he chose to eat Thai. He told me the only dish he likes is pad Thai. Pad Thai uses rice noodles, not wheat. The obvious solution was to take him off wheat products, and his gut symptoms resolved quickly.

Identifying your food sensitivities is like climbing a staircase. Sometimes you are spot on and you know exactly what foods affect you and other times you stumble or back step and have to start again. It can be hard like climbing a staircase, but not so hard that it can't be done or that you won't be rewarded at the end.

The light at the end of the tunnel is more energy, more focus, more clarity, less gas and bloating, less stomach pain, and better bowel movements. It's worth it, I promise.

IDENTIFYING FOOD SENSITIVITIES

How do you go about finding what your food sensitivities are and why call them sensitivities and not allergies?

Food allergies are when you react to the scratch test in your allergist's office. Allergists only identify an allergy if it displays a specific immunoglobulin reaction. Immunoglobulin...sounds like something you would find hiding in your bushes on halloween doesn't it? Immunoglobulins are cells of your immune system that react to different stimuli. They are the scouts that identify when there is a foreign invader and flag that invader for future destruction.

There are four types of immunoglobulins.

- IgA often relates to a reaction or inflammation at the intestinal lining.
- IgG is useful to identify food sensitivities that have a delayed reaction.

- IgE is the marker used to identify allergens.
- IgM is not used as often for food sensitivities. It is the first line of defense against infections.

Allergists only identify an allergy if it displays an IgE reaction. Functional medicine practitioners will use an IgG test, or other immunoglobulins, to screen for sensitivities. Sensitivities are reactions that can range from upset stomach to skin rashes and look and act very much like an allergy, but that term is reserved for allergists.

You can identify sensitivities in three ways.

1. You can get a blood test that looks for the immunoglobulin reaction. Although you will get some results that will show a false sensitivity (false positive) or a false absence of sensitivity (false negative) it is one of the more quantitative ways to evaluate a food sensitivity.
   At the time of this writing, Cyrex Labs is the only testing lab available to practicing doctors that screen for the myriad of gluten antibodies, not just alpha gliadin which is the only gluten marker that is typically tested.
2. You can use an "energy medicine" method, such as muscle testing or a sway test. This may or may not be in your belief system, but I have used muscle testing long enough that I trust it as a screening method. Muscle testing is when you put a substance on a person's body and identify if a strong muscle stays strong or goes weak when resistance is applied.

3. Elimination Diet. If you remove a food and the reaction resolves you are on the right track, but it is not foolproof. You have to avoid the food for an undetermined period of time and allow the body to heal. Often for at least two months without cheating. It may not be only one food. It may be more and you may still have symptoms until all the sensitivities are removed, such as dairy in addition to gluten. It can also be sneaky and you may find yourself ingesting your sensitivities without knowing it. An example would be gluten in lipstick. If you are celiac and highly sensitive to gluten, even the amount that is in lipstick can perpetuate your symptoms.

No need to be overwhelmed, you can contact a functional medicine practitioner to navigate this area with you.

The most common food sensitivities include:

- Dairy Products
- Gluten
- Peanuts
- Shellfish
- Eggs
- Corn
- Soy
- Coffee
- Alcohol

CHAPTER HIGHLIGHTS

★ Allergists only identify an allergy if it displays a specific immunoglobulin reaction.

★ Sensitivities are reactions that can range from upset stomach to skin rashes and look and act very much like an allergy.

Conclusion

Ready to Supercharge Your Lifestyle?

You don't have to slog through your day feeling fatigued or whip through your kitchen like a tornado, consuming everything you see when you get home from work. The Supercharged Method can help you live a happier, healthier lifestyle.

Brianne came to see me with the goal of losing weight. She was so frustrated and angry with herself. She had lost weight when she was younger, why not now? We identified foods that she was sensitive to, and she actively and dutifully avoided them. She was still not losing the fifty pounds she so desperately wanted to lose. I asked her if she was sticking to The Supercharged Method and she told me she was, until there was a cookie to try, or chips that happened to be on the counter. Yes, one hundred percent she was sticking to the program, except for all that.

I get it, I've been there too and sometimes still am. The difference is that I have found where on the spectrum of compliance I need to be to get the results I want, and I have figured out how to harness "why" I'm choosing to do it. The spectrum of compliance goes from doing everything by the book and checking it off as you go to doing the bare minimum needed to see results. It takes some work to figure out where you fall on the spectrum, but trust that you will find it. The spot on the spectrum probably isn't where it was when you were 20 or even 30, so now you need to reevaluate and rediscover what works for you.

Brianne was upset when she found out that she had to forgo her Tollhouse cookies before bed but regained a new sense of discovery when she found that by making her own cookies with ingredients that didn't set off inflammation, fatigue, and weight gain, she was so much happier. The Supercharged Method got her to her goal weight, the amazing way her body feels keeps her there.

You have all the tools you need to regain the energy clarity and focus you are looking for using The Supercharged Method. It may not always be easy but I promise you it will be worth it. Today is your day to not only feel amazing in your body right now but to know that you are on a path that decreases your risk for disease in your future.

I'm available to help you on your Supercharged journey! Learn more on my website www.thesuperchargedmethod.com. Or connect with me on social media.

Review Inquiry

Hey, it's Stacey here.

I hope you've enjoyed the book, finding it both useful and fun. I have a favor to ask you.

Would you consider giving it a rating wherever you bought the book? Online book stores are more likely to promote a book when they feel good about its content, and reader reviews are a great barometer for a book's quality.

So please go to the website of wherever you bought the book, search for my name and the book title, and leave a review. If able, perhaps consider adding a picture of you holding the book. That increases the likelihood your review will be accepted!

Many thanks in advance,

Dr. Stacey

Will You Share the Love?

Get this book for a friend, associate, or family member!

If you have found this book valuable and know others who would find it useful, consider buying them a copy as a gift. Special bulk discounts are available if you would like your whole team or organization to benefit from reading this. Just contact www.thesuperchargedmethod.com,
info@thesuperchargedmethod.com, or 248-213-1332.

Would You Like Dr. Stacey Francis to Speak to Your Organization?

Book Dr. Stacey Now!

Dr. Stacey accepts a limited number of speaking/coaching/training engagements each year. To learn how you can bring her message to your organization, call or email info@thesuperchargedmethod.com or 248-213-1332.

Contact

CONTACT DR. FRANCIS

I would love to hear your success stories using The Supercharged Method. You can contact me at:

info@thesuperchargedmethod.com

I'm available to help you on your Supercharged journey! Learn more on my website:

www.thesuperchargedmethod.com

Follow me on social media:

www.facebook.com/drstaceyfrancis

www.instagram.com/drstaceyfrancis

If you have a group that is looking for a fun and interactive speaker, contact our clinic.

The Supercharged Method Online Programs are coming soon and they are going to be awesome!! Stay tuned.

The Supercharged Method
RECAP

FIVE POWERFUL STEPS

There are five things you can do to have success in regaining energy and eliminating brain fog. The "how, why, where, and when" are in the previous chapters, but here are the basic steps:

1. Step 1: Prepare your home by removing energy-robbing and inflammatory foods and restocking your kitchen with energy-boosting and anti-inflammatory foods.
2. Step 2: Drink half your body weight in ounces of water daily.
3. Step 3: Get seven to nine hours of good sleep each night.
4. Step 4: Eat one serving of protein and two servings of vegetables every three to four hours in a 12 hour or less time frame.
5. Step 5: Set aside 20 minutes a day to relax and breathe.

THE BASICS OF The Supercharged Method

DRINK EIGHT GLASSES OF WATER A DAY

Raise your hand if getting eight glasses or 64 ounces of water in a day is just not happening? I understand. There are many reasons you may be drinking less water than you need. If you have a life where stopping to go to the bathroom is an inconvenience, you may choose to drink less. You may not feel thirsty if you are drinking coffee, cola, or eating instead of drinking water. And some people just have a hard time drinking water. I do understand...but you still have to drink water. Your "uncaffeinated, sugar-free, artificial-flavor-free and artificial-sweetener-free" water.

Plain water is:

- Calorie-free. It will not contribute to calories that you do not want and do not need.
- Sugar-free. It will not spike insulin and cause your blood sugar to be out-of-balance.
- Caffeine-free. It will not stimulate you, cause jitters, or cause a spike in cortisol.
- Chemical-free. It will not be a burden on your liver, kidneys, or gastrointestinal tract.
- Food Dye-free. It will not be a burden on your brain, causing loss of focus or clarity.

Drinking eight glasses or 64 ounces is the bare minimum. Half your body weight in ounces of water is more the rule. That means

64 ounces would be the amount for someone who weighs 128 pounds. How much do you weigh?

Your weight divided by two equals the amount of water in ounces that is recommended per day. More if you have been sweating.

If it seems overwhelming to go from drinking nothing all day to drinking half your body weight in ounces a day, start slower, but start somewhere and give yourself a goal of increasing the amount by four ounces every few days.

WHAT CONSTITUTES WATER BUT TASTES BETTER THAN WATER?

Here is a list of water alternatives if you just can't get yourself to embrace plain water.

- Decaffeinated herbal tea (any variety, hot or cold)
- Infused water with fruit, vegetables or herbs floating in it (flavors the water and can be removed before drinking)
- Water with lemon or lime juice and monk fruit, stevia, or another natural sugar-free sweetener
- Naturally sweetened, sugar-free electrolyte drink (eg. Ultima Replenisher or Waterdrop Microdrink)
- Naturally flavored, unsweetened (or naturally sweetened) carbonated water

MAKE IT A HABIT

There are many ways to track your water. From water tracking sheets where you cross off a box every time you drink your water to specialized apps and water bottles that remind you to drink water.

Starting early in the morning can help you reach your water goals. If you drink 32 ounces by lunch, you're halfway there. If you finish by dinner time, you can check the box for water intake for the day and give yourself a high-five. Not to mention, you won't be waking to run to the bathroom all night.

To get more information on why water is important and ideas to up your water game, see Section Three.

SLEEP SEVEN TO NINE RESTFUL HOURS

You know that you feel better when you obtain the right amount of restful sleep. You wake up with a clear head ready to take on the day. So many times we forfeit sleep for work, late night TV, or social media scrolling. Sometimes it's the inability to fall asleep or stay asleep.

It is time to make sleep a priority. Your brain and body will thank you for it. In fact, you will be even more productive and manage your time better when you steadily obtain good sleep.

Seven to nine hours of restful sleep and all your zzzz's provides these benefits:

- Better brain function
- Mood is more upbeat and stable
- Better blood pressure control
- Greater muscle repair
- Stronger immune system
- More stable blood sugar levels

Here are some quick tips that will be expanded upon in the sleep chapter.

1. Designate seven to nine hours that you will devote to sleeping, taking into account all the nighttime rituals you do before you get into bed. Changing your clothes, brushing your teeth, setting your alarm, and preparing for the next day all need to be done before your designated eight hours start.
2. Wind down. Take at least an hour to be without electronics, bright lights and loud noises prior to going to bed.
3. Finish eating three hours before bed, and go to sleep no later than three hours after you have eaten.
4. Take an epsom salt bath before bed.
5. Meditate.
6. Do restorative yoga.
7. Keep your room dark.
8. Move electronics, including your smartphone, into the hallway.
9. Use lavender essential oil, hemp oil, or melatonin if needed.

Once again, you can use a sleep tracker or a sleep app, if that helps.

There are many reasons for poor sleep. To learn the reasons some people can't sleep and what to do about it, see Section Four.

OWN YOUR EATING

Eat 1+2, EVERY 3–4 IN 12

"You never change things by fighting the existing reality.
To change something, build a new model that
makes the existing model obsolete."

—Richard Buckminster Fuller

1+2
Every 3-4
in 12

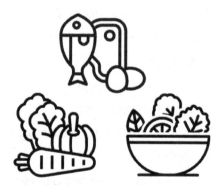

means...

1 serving of protein
plus
2 servings of vegetables
eaten every 3 to 4 hours,
in a 12 hour time frame.

PROTEIN + VEGETABLE + DIFFERENT VEGETABLE

EVERY 3–4 HOURS

IN A 12 HOUR OR LESS TIME PERIOD.

Can I make it any clearer? Protein is important. Eat it. Vegetables are important. Eat them. Allow your insulin to return to baseline by not snacking between meals, and rest your digestive tract for at least 12 hours.

To follow Mr. Fuller's quote above, you can change your way of eating by starting with great whole foods and eating them often enough that you are not craving the processed foods that make you sick. This is your new model that is so easy, delicious, and free of drama or deprivation that it will make your old way of eating obsolete.

Choose organic, grass-fed or wild-caught animal proteins.

Choose one serving of protein:		Choose one serving of a low glycemic vegetable:		Choose one serving of a different low glycemic vegetable:
Chicken	+	Asparagus	+	Artichoke
Fish	+	Broccoli	+	Brussels Sprouts
Beef	+	Cabbage	+	Celery
Bison	+	Cauliflower	+	Cucumber
Game or Organ Meat	+	Green Beans	+	Dark Greens (Spinach, Bok Choy..)
Eggs	+	Bell Peppers	+	Eggplant
Dairy	+	Zucchini	+	Mushroom

Choose one serving of protein:		Choose one serving of a low glycemic vegetable:		Choose one serving of a different low glycemic vegetable:
Soy	+	Yellow Squash	+	Okra
Nuts or Seeds	+	Seaweed or Dulse	+	Onion
Legumes...	+	Tomatoes...	+	Radish...

Eat one serving of protein <u>at every meal</u>.

Protein examples (organic, wild-caught, or grass-fed): chicken or other poultry, fish, beef, bison or other game and organ meats, lamb, shellfish, eggs, dairy, soy, nuts, seeds and legumes.

+

Eat at least two servings of low glycemic, above the ground, vegetables <u>at every meal</u>.

Low glycemic vegetable examples: asparagus, cabbage, mixed greens, broccoli, cauliflower, green beans, zucchini, yellow squash, etc.

A serving size of low glycemic or above the ground vegetables (not including corn) is half a cup to one cup.

Limit higher glycemic vegetables like corn and grains (bread, pasta, rice, and oats), below the ground vegetables like potatoes, parsnips, carrots, and beets and all fruit to two servings <u>a day</u>.

One serving equals half a cup of these higher glycemic foods.

Include a tablespoon of healthy fat per meal, or if you are having a larger serving of high-fat food like guacamole (Who can eat only one tablespoon of guacamole?! Not me.) then skip the fat serving in another meal.

Eat every three to four hours. That allows you to eat often enough that you are not skipping meals or reaching for something sugary because you are starving. The time also allows your insulin to come down before it rises again at your next meal.

Keep your eating window in a 12 hour, or less, time period. This lets your gastrointestinal system rest sufficiently, and once it completes digestion your body can digest other material, like bacteria and damaged cells, that is not needed. This is called autophagy. It is the body's way of removing damaged cells. If you are interested in knowing more about this function you can read the November 2018 study in the journal *Nature Reviews Cancer* which presents the mechanism of fasting induced autophagy.

Ultimately, eating this way gives your body plenty of food so you aren't starving or feeling deprived. You are eating whole foods that your body needs and loves. Reducing sugar or an abundance of high glycemic foods helps your blood sugar stay balanced and if you have a sweet tooth there are sugar alternatives that won't interfere with your goal of being supercharged.

Following the "1+2 every 3–4 in 12" plan is a doable lifestyle that is sustainable.

A SAMPLE DAY MAY LOOK LIKE THIS:

Water after waking and between meals, and herbal tea until the first meal.

10 a.m.: Eggs + mushrooms + spinach sauteed in 1T butter with ½ cup mixed berries.

1 p.m.: Tuna + romaine + red pepper with 1T olive oil dressing and ½ cup quinoa.

4 p.m.: Hummus + red peppers + cucumbers and 3 brazil nuts (nuts can count as a fat or a protein).

7 p.m.: Grilled chicken + broccoli + asparagus and ½ cup baked potato with 1T butter and a small baked apple.

Herbal tea after dinner

20 MINUTES OF SELF CARE

Support your adrenal glands and prevent burnout by giving yourself 20 minutes of self care.

Self care is relaxing and restorative. It is not watching the news or a horror movie. The point is to slow your heart rate and your breathing, relax your muscles and think good thoughts.

Meditate or pray. Let your mind go blank to give your brain and body a time out. This can ground you and renew you. You might just notice you can focus and concentrate more after 20 minutes of meditation or prayer.

Deep breathe. Allow your lungs to expand fully and then push out all the air. This helps with adrenal function and anxiety. Breathe in for a count of four, hold for a count of four, breathe out for a count of four and then hold for a count of four. Do four cycles then relax for a few minutes.

Stretch your muscles. Do it gently. I know all you yogis out there can bend and twist until you could contend for a spot in Cirque du Soleil. That is not the goal. Slowly start stretching, and as soon as you start to feel the stretch, do not go past it. Stay in that position until the sensation completely disappears before you move any further into the stretch. Go slow and pay attention. Breathe into your muscles and allow them to relax.

Walk. This does not mean power walk. It means stroll. Weight-bearing, low impact and easy on your joints, walking is restorative movement.

Say nice things. Your words are powerful. No one expected Japanese scientist Dr. Masaru Emoto to leave a mark like he did. He photographed two samples of water. One sample he yelled at and spoke unkindly to, the other he spoke soft and lovingly to. Under the microscope the images of the hated water were scrambled and disorganized. The loved water was symmetrical and organized. Keep that in mind when you talk to yourself and others.

Draw, sing, write, read, hug, or take a bath. There are so many ways to self care. It should calm you down, slow your breathing, and relax you. Pick the one that works for you.

RUN LABS

If you are a person who gets yearly blood draws you are ahead of the game. Your doctor is making sure that you will be treated if you develop a disease or disease process. This is good, but it could be great. I call this sick care or disease management if they are checking your blood work yearly and waiting for the values to land outside of the conventional lab range to treat you. These doctors rarely recommend diet improvements or lifestyle changes—not because they don't think they are helpful (although there are those who don't) but because they are wait-ing for you to request them. At that point, they might guide you, or refer you to a nutritional or lifestyle specialist. That is what I consider "good."

There are also doctors who will acknowledge that there are lab ranges and optimal or functional lab ranges. These are typically narrow ranges that indicate you are functioning at your best and that you are "on point" with your nutrition, sleep, stress, choices, behaviors, habits, and genetic expression. They know if you are between lab range and optimal range there are things you can do to improve your health and prevent disease. This is truly health care, and doctors who take measures to help you prevent disease are "great."

The Supercharged Method is not intended to be used without a health practitioner's oversight. If you are out of lab range, that is the territory that your licensed health practitioner should address. They have spent years evaluating and navigating the intricacies of blood work. Rely on them to help you resolve any values that are out of range.

The Supercharged Method is specifically, and only, for the ranges that lie between lab range and optimal range. If you order your own blood work and find a test that your doctor doesn't normally run is out of range, you need to have them help you bring it back into lab range. You can do The Supercharged Method alongside that treatment.

There are different ways to identify a health problem. Symptoms are one, labs are another. Not just any labs. The right labs. Although the labs I'm suggesting are not an extensive list, they are the ones that, when in optimal range, make the most difference. For a more thorough look at labs, see Section Four.

If you have a health condition, such as iron deficiency anemia, your blood work will show enough abnormality to alert your doctor. An out of lab range would be indicated by an "H" or "L" on your lab report. The process of your labs moving out of optimal range may be missed if treatment only occurs once you are out of range. You can have symptoms for years (which doesn't mean you have a condition, but it could indicate the makings of one) as you move from optimal health to lower and lower iron levels before the values of your blood work show you are out of range.

We need to look more thoroughly every time blood work is performed, and not just look at whether the levels are in range or not, but how they are moving. Are you barely in range and slowly moving back into a healthy range or more out of range? Let's catch it then, before there are symptoms and before it's a problem that takes more work to correct.

The following are the labs you can look at to evaluate markers for The Supercharged Method.

You may request it from your doctor or use a lab on your own. They cover blood sugar, anemias, thyroid, and inflammation.

Blood Sugar:

- Glucose
- Insulin
- Hemoglobin A1c
- Triglycerides

Thyroid:

- Mean corpuscular hemoglobin
- Hemoglobin
- Hematocrit
- Methylmalonic acid

Anemias:

- Ferritin
- Iron
- Total iron binding capacity
- Mean corpuscular volume
- Thyroid stimulating hormone
- Total thyroxine
- Free thyroxine
- Total triiodothyronine
- Free triiodothyronine
- Reverse triiodothyronine
- Thyroperoxidase antibody
- Thyroglobulin antibody

Inflammation:

- C-reactive protein
- Fibrinogen
- Erythrocyte sedimentation rate
- Homocysteine
- 25 hydroxy vitamin D

Testimonials

"In 2019, I developed a nasty digestive issue, following a period on a full spectrum antibiotic for a sinus infection. I experienced intense bloating, gas, and abdominal pain after eating. It usually lasted through the night, making it difficult and sometimes impossible to sleep. Even when I did sleep I was often exhausted the next day. I don't know what I would have done without the help of Dr. Francis. She suggested a SIBO test, and when it came back positive, she set me on the road to recovery with a restrictive diet, some really effective supplements, and all the emotional support I needed. I am now able to eat a normal diet without any problems. Dr. Francis' program has not only helped with these digestive issues, but in some ways I feel better than I did before this digestive problem. I am more energetic, and the frequent heartburn issues I had also seem to have gone away."

—Diana Munch

"Since working with Dr. Stacey my energy levels have increased. I'm able to stand for longer periods of time without achy legs, digestion is much better, and brain fog is gone. Prior to seeing her I couldn't work out without feeling drained and with extreme muscle soreness. The opposite is true now. She has been a godsend to me!"

—Andrea Walker

"After completing the 10-Day Supercharged Cleanse, I've noticed that my brain fog is gone, and I feel energized. Even though I consider my usual diet to be pretty healthy overall, I've noticed that perhaps I don't always get adequate amounts of protein, which leads me to indulge in cravings easily around 5:00 p.m. During the cleanse, I never felt hungry, which allowed me to notice that I can sometimes crave sweet things out of habits or to avoid doing unpleasant tasks. The cleanse gave me the opportunity to reset and increase my awareness of my current habits to make the necessary adjustments. Thank you Dr. Stacey and team."

—Marie Thouvenot

"Dr. Stacey, I wanted to take a moment to thank you for this amazing and revealing cleanse experience. I did not execute it absolutely perfectly (at times), but even so, the results were quite astonishing. Let me first say that I am a menopausal woman. Why does that matter? I found out that the strength of my hot flashes is in direct proportion to what I eat. NOT having sugar, alcohol, and any processed foods DRASTICALLY cut down on the intensity of the...power surges. I also started sleeping through the night. THIS. This is miraculous. And healing. With not snacking between meals, I also started listening to my body more and eating for all the right reasons. Finally, and this was most important to me, my mind had amazing clarity. You don't realize how foggy and fuzzy you were until you're not anymore. Thank you so much for providing this opportunity and new way of relating with food. You are deeply appreciated."

—Julie Steinmayer

"In order to express my reaction to the ten-day cleanse with Dr. Stacey, I need to provide some background. About four years ago I began the ketogenic diet that was recommended for one of my children. I did it to encourage and support my child's health. I do not know how much weight I lost because I did not believe in scales, but I went from wearing a size 16/18 to a size six/eight. I did not feel hungry or restricted. I kept this weight off until about a year into the Pandemic. Sitting home all day, working remotely created habits of eating all day at my desk. In the past nine months I have tried many ways to get healthy again. I have been experiencing joint pain, migraines, lower back pain, fatigue, and the like. I found with the various diets and mind sets, that I was not able to make the progress that I was looking for. It was around this time that Dr. Stacey Francis mentioned that she was going to be offering a ten-day cleanse. I told her immediately that I wanted to participate. However, that was three weeks before the cleanse. This timing created two situations for me. On the one hand, I gave myself the freedom to eat anything I wanted, in any amount at any time. As freeing as that was, I did not find myself satiated or satisfied, just full and bloated. The other situation was time. I had three weeks to mentally prepare myself for a change.

Dr. Stacey scheduled the cleanse to begin on a Wednesday. In preparation, I used the weekend to cook a variety of proteins using the approved foods and portions. I also prepped vegetables. When Wednesday arrived, my head was in the plan and I was ready to go. Dr. Stacey provided me with all of the necessary supplements and tools to proceed. In addition she hosted a nightly zoom session that created community and provided support and learning opportunities. The cleanse was originally scheduled to last ten days with an option to extend for an additional ten days. By the end of the first ten days I lost 8.6 pounds, had no cravings for sugar, caffeine, or alcohol, and never felt hungry.

In addition to the loss of toxins and weight, I did notice some other benefits. As a person that has fought with migraines for over 15 years, I take a monthly injection to prevent them and additional medications when the migraines break through. I was unable to fill these prescriptions due to new year policy confusion and I went six weeks without the injections or a migraine. This is a major life changer for me. I also noticed that I had no joint pain. I have been taking medications for shoulder and neck problems as well. I have had no discomfort and am looking to wean off these medications as I continue through the detox.

This has been, and I expect will continue to be, an amazing experience. I have learned that I have control of what I eat, I can eat only when hungry and be done when satisfied. Participating in this cleanse with Dr. Stacey has put me back in control of my well being, which I will forever be grateful for."

3 month update

"As of March 19, I have been off of my Aimovig injections for 3 months which means it is completely out of my system. I can honestly report that my migraine/headaches are few and far between and quite manageable. I used to report 3+ migraines per week and have less than that per month now. In addition, I'm quickly able to determine the cause of the migraine, which gives me control over them in the future. If that wasn't enough, which it is, I'm also down 18.8 pounds."

—Debi Banooni

Dr. Stacey offered an opportunity to join in a ten-day cleanse. I was reluctant but then I thought this is a great opportunity because Dr. Stacey did all the work to get it ready. I can do this. Not only was Dr. Stacey an incredible leader, supportive, and informative but she made this a fun experience. I learned so much more than I expected. I have gained a lot of confidence in my ability to maintain a significantly healthier lifestyle and it is sustainable. I was never hungry. I would recommend this to anyone who needs a restart. It wasn't all easy but the good stuff usually requires effort and the rewards far outway the challenges. Dr. Stacey will help you with the hurdles. Thank you for this experience. Going forward I hope to educate my family and help them learn life long habits for vitality and health.

—Beth Bradford

"Dr. Francis' Supercharged Cleanse was beneficial in helping to plan a new approach to eating clean. The great communication and frequent information were extremely helpful in planning a new lifestyle. The team approach during the program was very supportive and provided encouragement throughout the day. The benefits I received were consistency, thoughtfulness, and planning that helped to contribute to an increased food awareness. Dr. Francis was readily available to respond to questions that arose. The program also incorporated more than food awareness. It incorporated meditation, deep breathing, and exercise to balance the clean eating. I would highly recommend this program for people wanting to start weight loss as well as improve their overall eating and health!"

—Vicki Astell

"Before the Supercharged Cleanse program began, I warned my family and co-workers that I may not be at my best and please give me a pass during the ten-day program. I have been pleasantly surprised that I did not turn into a monster; I had more food to eat than I could handle, and I felt wonderful! I have more energy and a huge sense of accomplishment for staying true to the program. Walking past sweets and treats is very easy now and only eating the four meals is food enough. My sleeping has improved so when I wake in the morning, I feel well rested. I enjoyed this program and have benefitted so much that I am continuing for an additional ten days. Bravo to Dr. Stacey and her staff for making this a wonderful, educational, and worthwhile program. I would do this program again."

—Robyn Flam

"I thought that the Supercharged Cleanse was one of the best things I've ever done for my health. I feel much better, I have more energy, and I'm empowered to take better care of myself. I am looking forward to the next 50 years and I think the Supercharged Cleanse has a lot to do with that."

—Bridget Kastl

"The Supercharged Cleanse was a great experience. Dr. Stacey and Jill did a great job making us feel comfortable and preparing us and it was absolutely doable. The foods were delicious and nutritious and we had so much support from all the members of the group on Facebook. We shared recipes and supported each other. This way of eating has become part of my lifestyle. I highly recommend it."

—Sue Carter

I have participated in and completed half a dozen detox/cleanse programs over the past decade. Most proved very challenging and difficult to finish. Dr. Stacey's Supercharged Cleanse is in a class by itself. I found her program easy to follow, easy to commit to and easy to complete. After the initial detoxing experiences, I wound up losing seven pounds in ten days and sleeping better at night. It is the complete package and I will absolutely revisit this program throughout the year. Thanks Dr. Stacey!

—Linda Charter

Following Dr. Stacey's eating plan has been such a positive experience for me. Two big wins were kicking my life-long caffeine habit and my "snacking hour," which I had established when my kids were little—I would mindlessly eat with them after school. Additionally, I have not felt bloated or had indigestion. This is something I was suffering with daily for about eight years!

Working with Dr. Francis and following her plan has given me control over my eating habits and given me the tools to continue to see success with my health. I feel liberated from my old habits and look forward to living my life healthfully.

— Jill McDonnell

I have been seeing Dr. Stacey for over six years. She provides excellent comprehensive wellness care. I recently completed her 2022 10-Day Supercharged Cleanse and I have to say it was incredible. A few benefits I experienced with this cleanse are: lost weight, less bloating/puffiness, clearer skin, better sleep, less brain fog, no sugar/salt cravings, much less joint pain and less inflammation. She provided everything needed to succeed on this plan and I highly recommend it!

— Mary Lynn Williams

Join our amazing community and get the health results you are looking for at www.thesuperchargedmethod.com

About the Author

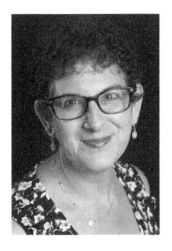

For over 25 years, Dr. Stacey Francis has been treating patients using chiropractic kinesiology and nutrition. As an expert in her field, she is an advocate for educating others in the brilliance of the human body. From neck pain to stomach pain, autoimmune disorders to allergies, Dr. Stacey serves the tired, frustrated, hopeless, and hurting, helping her patients achieve optimal wellness through balancing the structural, biochemical, and psyche systems of the body.

Dr. Stacey received her Doctorate from the National College of Chiropractic in Illinois and maintains an active membership with the Michigan Association of Chiropractors. She is an experienced public speaker and has presented for General Motors, Oakland County of Michigan, Verizon Media, InForum, Brightwing and many religious institutions and corporations. In addition, she is a published author, has appeared multiple times on Fox 2 News, and has taught anatomy and physiology at the Beaumont School of Yoga Therapy.

Dr. Stacey has lived in and served the metro Detroit area for over 29 years with her husband, two sons, and their poogle, Spencer. When not doing the thing she loves most (working), she can be found wandering art galleries, art fairs, farmer's markets, dancing, drawing, cooking, or shopping at her favorite place on earth, Trader Joe's.

Dr. Stacey Francis can be reached at:
www.thesuperchargedmethod.com

Made in the USA
Middletown, DE
13 October 2022

12604910R00205